THE UNDIET

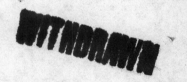

Albert R. Marston, Ph.D., is a professor of psychology and psychiatry at the University of Southern California. Widely published in the field of weight control, Dr. Marston and his work have been discussed in such popularly acclaimed magazines as *U.S. News and World Report, Glamour, House and Garden,* and *Bon Appetit.* He has worked with thousands of overweight people, is a well-known lecturer on the topic of weight control, and has appeared numerous times on radio and TV talk shows.

THE UNDIET

A Psychological Approach to Permanent Weight Control

Albert R. Marston, Ph.D.

A SPECTRUM BOOK

Prentice-Hall, Inc., Englewood Cliffs, New Jersey 07632

Library of Congress Cataloging in Publication Data

Marston, Albert R.
    The undiet.

    "A Spectrum Book."
    Bibliography: p.
    Includes index.
    1. Reducing—Psychological aspects.   I. Title.
RM222.2.M363   1983   613.2'5'019   82-21417
ISBN 0-13-936815-9
ISBN 0-13-936807-8 (pbk.)

This book is available at a
special discount when ordered in bulk quantities. For
information, contact Prentice-Hall, Inc., General Publishing
Division, Special Sales, Englewood Cliffs, N.J. 07632

A SPECTRUM BOOK

10 9 8 7 6 5 4 3 2 1

Printed in the United States of America

ISBN 0-13-936807-8 (PBK.)

ISBN 0-13-936815-9

Editorial and production supervision
by Ethel Waters and Cyndy Lyle Rymer
Manufacturing buyer Christine Johnston
Cover design by Hal Siegel

Prentice-Hall International, Inc., London
Prentice-Hall of Australia Pty. Limited, Sydney
Prentice-Hall of Canada Inc., Toronto
Prentice-Hall of India Private Limited, New Delhi
Prentice-Hall of Japan, Inc., Tokyo
Prentice-Hall of Southeast Asia Pte. Ltd., Singapore
Whitehall Books Limited, Wellington, New Zealand
Editora Prentice-Hall do Brasil, Ltda., Rio de Janeiro

CONTENTS

APPENDIX/196

INDEX/215

PREFACE
FOR PROFESSIONALS

(For dieticians, home economists, physical educators, nutritionists, counselors, chiropractors, physicians, psychologists, nurses, health educators, physical therapists, and other weight control specialists)

The Undiet is written for the layperson who wishes to combine a diet (or modified fast) and/or calorie counting with a behavior modification program to effect long-term weight control. It is also designed as a framework for professionals to use in setting up weight control programs, or for teachers (for example, at the community college level) who would like to supplement their courses with a practical weight control program as an experiential learning technique.

The Appendix is designed to guide the layperson in setting up an *Undiet Club* as a support group for weight loss and maintenance. We believe that the self-run group is a cost-effective way to bridge the gap between the printed program and the professional. In busy institutional settings and private practices, the professional can serve as consultant to such groups and as a primary referral for group members presenting special problems. These groups can be used as the sole treatment for mild or moderately uncomplicated cases of overweight. Severe or morbidly obese patients could be monitored periodically by a professional while using the Undiet Club as an ongoing support system.

We hope that this book is general enough for use by all professionals helping overweight people and specific enough to be a complete guide for the overweight person. We would appreciate feedback from you about your experience using the book.

ACKNOWLEDGMENTS

The Undiet is based on my knowledge accumulated over many years of helping overweight people. Much of this work involved collaboration with my wife, Marlene Marston, Ph.D. who has made major contributions to the content, style, and organization of the material. Some of the material appeared in articles in *Slimming* magazine in Great Britain with the collaboration of then editor Audrey Eyton, in our course Correspondence Weight Reduction, and in our jointly written audio cassette program, *Comprehensive Weight Control*, 1980 (BMA, 200 Park Avenue South, New York, New York, 10003). I would like to acknowledge staff and students and colleagues who made many contributions to the work. I am especially grateful to the clients themselves whose knowledge about the problems of being overweight have been shared with one another and with us. This book reflects what I have learned from them as well as what I have taught.

I would like to acknowledge the special contribution of my son, Joshua Marston, for his creation of the title, *The Undiet*.

INTRODUCTION

The Undiet has several features that make it unique, including the basic concept that recognizes the importance of integrating the use of diets or fasting with behavior modification to solve the psychological and social problems surrounding the control of eating.

The *Partner Participation Program* is introduced at the end of Chapter 3. We recognize that many readers live with someone, whether spouse, other family members, or roommate(s). The partner participation program not only helps the reader to deal with problems involved in group living situations, but shows how to harness the help available from the people living with him/her.

Another special feature of *The Undiet* involves the issue of help outside the home. The author has conducted groups and other programs to assist overweight people. I am convinced that group support can be very helpful in any difficult process of personal change. However, the group need not be a costly, professionally run effort. In fact, there is some evidence that the more involved the participants are in running the group, the more successful they will be. Therefore, we are advocating the establishment of *Undiet Clubs*, made up of overweight people who meet regularly to help one another by using the principles presented in this book and sharing solutions to problems they have in common.

I hope that you will take the initiative to find or set up such a group in your area. You can use a community center bulletin board, free announcements in local or school newspapers or on radio stations, listings in church bulletins, regular community recreation or education programs, and many other resources to set up an *Undiet Club*. A dietician, home economics teacher, or other professional may be available to help you get started. You can meet in free rooms available in the community, or at one another's homes. I have written a special Appendix at the end of the book to guide you in setting up and operating an *Undiet Club*. I hope that you will take advantage of this idea. The effort you make to find or form a club will pay off in many ways—motivation of involvement in a group, help and support from others, and, perhaps most important, the satisfaction of being of help to others.

chapter one
GETTING OFF THE DIET MERRY-GO-ROUND

"I'll tell you what I'm going to do, ladies and gentlemen; step right up and get the latest miracle cure, our magical, mysterious new method to lose weight quickly and painlessly.

"You say you've heard it all before. You've just gotten off another ride on the diet merry-go-round. You've been on grapefruit for fourteen days, ate a whole side of beef, drank gallons of water, fasted with protein liquids, protein powders, protein shampoo. The pounds disappeared magically and reappeared the same way."

You say you're fed up with diets (sorry!); at least until the next best-seller comes along. "There must be a better way," you say. "Where's the wonder drug the *National Enquirer* keeps promising us? You know, the one where you eat ten thousand calories a day, but somehow they sneak through your body untouched and disappear, leaving you satisfied but svelte."

If you're seriously overweight, you may be desperately considering intestinal bypass surgery, or having your jaws wired shut, or moving into a residential treatment program for six months.

If you're reading this book, you have the suspicion, if not the complete conviction, that your problem with weight is in your head as well as in the rest of your body. You may have lost weight and regained it many times. You may even be at your goal weight

1

right now. Why does the problem persist? Could psychology hold the answer, the magic that will allow you to think yourself thin or fantasize your way to a really new body? We wish that we could tell you that if you understood how your mother, or your love life, or the way you hold your fork causes you to be overweight, your body would shrink more than your head.

At the risk of having you put this book down, or even not buy it, we must state up front, clearly and emphatically, that we have not discovered "the cure." We will not reveal a secret formula which, if followed to the letter, will lead you down the path to the paradise of a permanently slim body. We don't want this to crush your hopes. But we do want you to be skeptical, not gullible. If you're a dieter of any rank, you've bought the promises of many would-be gurus. It's time for you to be skeptical and hard-nosed and to demand that any new approach be sensible and deliver meaningful results.

Having said that we don't have *the* answer, we want to say, just as emphatically, that we do have a lot of different answers. This book will help you to understand your problems in new ways; more important, it will guide you with concrete suggestions toward permanent improvement in your self-control of eating.

IT'S NOT A PROBLEM
BUT MANY PROBLEMS

Some experts estimate that over forty million Americans are overweight. Many more are either on their way up or have reached a shaky goal weight and await the near certainty of regaining. These millions probably share only one thing in common: When they are gaining weight, they consume more calories than they burn. It's unlikely that there is one obese personality or one behavior pattern which, if changed, will cure or prevent obesity. You are as different from your fellow overweight sufferer as you are from the glamorous thin models who grace the covers of our magazines. In fact, it is likely that the model shares your eating control problem just as much as your currently overweight cousin.

*Non*overweight people binge, gorge, eat too fast, skip breakfast, avoid exercise, eat junk food—they do all the things you try to hide from. The last sentence, if you were not already aware of it, may be making you very angry. "Then why me?" you may be silently screaming. Many overweight people, and some respected scientists, are very caught up in this question. Maybe it's your genes, your hormones, or your fate. We can't be sure, but we are sure that you have lots of company and that until something better comes along, your control of your eating and exercise is still the only route to permanent weight management. That's frustrating to accept. We know because we've both lost weight (less than many of you and more than many), and we know that losing it was the *beginning* of achieving control, not the *end*. We don't feel as if we have some incurable disease, but for whatever social, psychological, and biological reasons, we are vulnerable to gaining weight. Having accepted that reality, we have tried to devise—for ourselves and for the thousands of our clients of past programs—an approach that makes weight control not only possible but tolerable. Yes, there are sacrifices; yes, there is hard work. But there is also a great deal of enjoyment of food and, above all, much satisfaction in our sense of self-control. We will, in this book, tell you what psychology has to offer you in achieving greater self-control of eating, as well as pass on to you the benefits of our own and our clients' experience. We have said that there is no one problem common to all overweight people and, therefore, no one solution for all of you. However, we believe that there are some problems, some principles, and some techniques that apply to most of you. There is as well an array of methods from which you can choose once you are aware of them and know more about yourself.

Therefore, this book will take two approaches. We will discuss principles and techniques that we feel are useful to most readers, and we will provide you with a way to choose a coordinated program of techniques best suited for you. Each chapter will discuss a problem area, give concrete advice, and outline specific things to do to solve that set of problems. You can go step by step through the book, trying the techniques and selecting the ones that work best for you, or you can look over the chapter headings and read selectively on the problems you may already know are especially relevant to you.

Before we begin with a more detailed analysis of the varied problems confronting the person who wants to improve eating control, we would like to set out briefly a few general principles which reflect our orientation and biases. These principles will be repeated and clarified many times through the book and will have their fullest meaning when we review them in the last chapter, .after you have applied them yourself.

DON'T BELIEVE ANY
GENERALIZATIONS ABOUT EATING
AND OBESITY, NOT EVEN THESE

Obesity is more society's fault than yours. Every overweight person, and anyone struggling with the problem of overweight, should have a good look around and understand how we are victims. This book focuses on how you can help yourself, but we feel that it's important to start out knowing where to put the blame. Overweight people add to their already heavy burden a sense of guilt and weakness. This image is often promoted by the nonoverweight who are only a slim majority of the population and who are likely themselves to succumb to the problem at some time in their lives. Here's where the blame belongs: food manufacturers who promote sweet and salty baby foods to hook helpless children; advertisers who spend billions of dollars to saturate the media with promotions of high-calorie foods; the industrial system, which has enmeshed most of us in boring and sedentary work; television, which provides us with a barrage of messages about food while we sit inactively hypnotized for twenty or thirty hours a week; the automobile industry, which gives us handy transportation down the block and to the supermarket; and on and on. We are cogs in an industrial wheel that has moved us from an active, low-stress life, fueled by wholesome natural foods, to our current state of inactivity and consumption of convenience foods. That you have shown the results of this change by being overweight rather than by having ulcers, high blood pressure, depression, or any of the myriads of other modern-day ills is probably more a matter of chance than choice.

To make matters worse, while you are enticed, pushed, and stressed toward your present overweight condition, you also are told to be thin to be healthy and beautiful—Catch-22 with a vengeance. It's no wonder that one result of this mess has been the emergence of Fat Liberation to join the ranks of the rebellious and the radical. These groups say that fat is beautiful and even healthy, that it is time for overweight people to stop struggling and to accept—even enjoy—the inevitable.

Despite the occasional confusing medical report which hints that being overweight may not be so bad, we still see more evidence that not being overweight is healthier. Nevertheless, the point of this attack on the social causes of overeating and underexercising, in addition to helping you wipe our unnecessary guilt, is to let you know that even if you win your personal battle, the war for your children's and grandchildren's health will have to be fought in the economic and political arena.

The awareness of the social nature of your problem also should help you to reexamine your goals in trying to control your weight. In the long run, you may want to evaluate not only your eating, but your whole recreational and occupational life-style, to discover what changes are open to you. While now you want to consider your goal weight in terms of your health and appearance criteria, before long you may shift your focus to such issues as nutrition, fitness, stress management, and the choice of a more satisfying life-style. For this reason, we will not simply suggest goal weights; instead, we will present many of our suggestions for change in a context which we hope will have broader usefulness to you than seeing changes on the bathroom scale.

Diets are okay. Having made fun of some of the many fad diets that have appeared over the years, we must make one stark fact of nature clear: To lose weight, you must eat less and/or increase your activity. All the psychological insights and life-style changes will help, but they will not directly lead to weight loss. You can control food intake by monitoring calories and knowing about nutrition and portion sizes. We think that this is ultimately the most lasting method for permanent control, and we will show you how to do this simply and comfortably. In the past we insisted that our clients avoid crash diets and to lose weight slowly by small changes in calorie intake and energy output. For some people, this is the most effective approach. However, we are increasingly aware that many overweight people, especially if the amount to be lost is relatively large, feel very frustrated with the slow-but-sure method. They need faster losses to feel enough progress and to keep from giving up. For this reason a diet, or a controlled fasting program, may be an important part of your weight-loss efforts. We will discuss selection of diets and the pitfalls involved, but the important point to remember at this stage is that a diet is not the solution to your weight problem. A diet can be a useful tool for weight loss, even weight maintenance, if used sensibly and integrated into a broader program of change.

Eating less is not fun. Any weight-loss effort involves depriving yourself of some of the pleasures of food that you have been used to since early childhood. For most people, deprivation is unpleasant, particularly if food has been an especially large part of the pleasure in your life. You can minimize the effects of the deprivation by telling yourself that it's only for a short time. But for those with a lot of weight to lose, this ploy won't help; for all of us, maintaining a lower weight will require a lifelong pattern of eating less quantity. We will focus on a number of principles and techniques to help with this problem. The general philosophy we propose has two parts: 1) the search for increased pleasure—physical, mental, and even spiritual—in other areas of your life to compensate for loss of eating pleasure, and 2) shifting the pleasure of eating from quantity to quality. Above all, it's important to minimize guilt and self-punishment and to try to be good to yourself while you're doing difficult tasks.

The sum of the parts is more than the whole. Eating, overeating, or being more active cannot be understood or changed by viewing the process as a simple act of will. There are several important areas that will be examined in later chapters in detail. They are:

1. Motivation doesn't go up or down by chance. Motivation is commitment to change. This commitment can be reinforced and maintained systematically.
2. Although we often eat alone, eating is an interpersonal event and is determined by our relationship with other people.

3. Eating means more to us than biological survival. Whether by learning or by instinct, we have come to associate eating with other emotions—increased pleasure; decreased tension, depression, or pain.
4. We often eat without awareness, quickly, automatically, and without real satisfaction. Gaining greater awareness of the process of eating will increase both pleasure and control.
5. Old habits die hard and require new habits to replace them. To acquire and strengthen habits requires practice and reward. Eventually your new habits may become easy, like riding a bike. Tolerating the shakiness and the falls is an important part of the learning process, as is learning from our own mistakes.

Problem solving is the key to success. Since we believe that the control of weight is a multifaceted problem, we are convinced that the only permanent solution is flexibility and an openness to looking at problems and trying many possible solutions in order to find what works best for that situation at that time.

Maintenance is more important than weight loss. This is implied in much of what we have said, but can't be emphasized too often. Old stresses continue; new ones come up. You must accept that no solution is permanent, that small failures are bound to happen, and that recovering from failure with minimum damage is the only reasonable goal in this lifelong process.

Getting help and giving help may be crucial. You are reading this book for help. You may have gone to groups or programs or professionals for help with your weight problem. People who seem to be doing it alone often are getting a great deal of help and support. It's important to view getting timely help as appropriate and not as a sign of weakness. You may accomplish a great deal with the methods we will be showing you, but you may find it important to link these methods to other sources of help. It is especially important during maintenance to accept the reality of our own vulnerability and to look for help—either old or new—when we need it. The balance between independence and stubborn pride is an important one.

The flip side to this principle involves the value in helping others. We have found that successful weight maintenance is often found in those people who help a friend or even become involved with a larger group of people working on similar problems.

These seven general principles introduce you to our philosophy and approach to the problem of weight control. The chapters that follow discuss these principles and suggest specific techniques for a variety of the problems involved in weight control. It's important that you use this book not only as a source of information, but also as a stimulus to take active steps in developing your own program of change. *Don't just wait for the next diet!*

HOW TO USE THIS BOOK

You could read through this book just as you would any other self-help or diet book and you would, we believe, gain a great deal of knowledge. We would like you to consider an alternative approach. Consider this your own independent weight-control program, to be carried out systematically over the next couple of months. After you've read the next two chapters, take a week to do the activities suggested. Choose a diet, if that's to be your strategy, and get used to keeping a diary on the convenient form we provide. After that, read a chapter a week, continuing the techniques that work well for you and adding new ones as you go along. By the end of the book you may not yet be at your goal weight, but you will have acquired a good array of tools to sharpen and use.

chapter two
MOTIVATION IS THE KEY

You may feel that you know a lot of things to do, but you just can't seem to stick to a diet or a program. This experience is often described as "I just don't seem to have the motivation." The solution to this problem is not simple, and it can't be found by looking for some special magic or new trick, or by finding someone to take you in hand and give you the proverbial "kick in the pants." Like any other problem, you've got to analyze it, work on the way you think about it, and then take some action to solve it.

We would like to describe several steps to take which will help you to understand your motivation and effectively increase it to develop control over your weight.

The first step in understanding motivation is to realize that the word is an umbrella term that includes more than one condition within us. One use of the term refers to all the physiological responses that drive or direct our behavior toward some goal: sexual arousal, hunger, thirst, fear, anger. One of the aspects of eating problems concerns the recognition of true hunger and the crossover of emotions—that is, eating to reduce fear or anger. This is discussed in detail in Chapter 9. These physiological responses also can drive or direct you to lose weight. For example, fear of a heart attack can lead you to lose weight, as can anger at a spouse who criticizes you for being fat. So, emotions can be motivating.

Important considerations in the use of emotion as motivation are the strength of the emotion and the availability of responses to reach the desired goal. For example, one well-known research project looked at the effect on cigarette smokers of showing people films about lung cancer. Two results are important for you. First, if the fear induced by the films is too strong, it backfires. If you are overwhelmed by fear, there is a tendency to avoid the issue altogether or to say, in effect, "Oh, what's the use!" Second, whether the fear directs you to change depends on the availability of a set of responses to effect the change. We have had clients who have said that they were learning a lot from our lectures, but that they didn't feel motivated enough at that time to lose weight. Then later we heard from them that some event scared them into doing something. It may have been a medical warning from a physician or a threat to a love relationship. At that point, when emotion was aroused, the resulting motivation could be harnessed to the skills learned during the lectures, and an effective and self-directed weight-loss program completed.

Another use of the term *motivation* refers to the thoughts we have about goals, the desire to reach them, the reasons for reaching them, and the expectation or hope that they will be reached. Some of the exercises we will be suggesting later in this chapter are designed to help you explore your reasons for losing weight. But first we would like you to consider some general issues about yourself and how they relate to your motivation to lose weight.

Motivation is often associated with the word *why*. For that question to be valuable, it has to lead to answers that can be dealt with. There is a tendency to ask the *why* questions in a way that explains our problems either in terms of the distant past or in terms of labels. Let's try to get beyond this kind of unproductive *why*. If I ask you, "Why are you overweight?" you might come up with answers like: "It's a sickness I have," "I was born with the tendency to be fat," "I am neurotic," "I am a compulsive eater," "I have no willpower," or "I just love food." Any or all of these answers could be correct, but they don't do you much good in your effort to change. They are answers that reduce motivation to lose weight and increase motivation to stay the same. However, you can try to set these answers aside. Here are a few thoughts that may help you ignore these unproductive explanations.

Millions of people are overweight. There is no evidence that more than a tiny percentage of them has a physical illness that causes obesity. There *are* a few diseases that contribute to obesity, and you would be wise to have a thorough examination by your physician to help you to set aside the illness answer to the *why* question.

Whether you are biologically predisposed to being fat is a factor that is difficult to determine. While it's true that obesity tends to run in families, it's also true that families tend to perpetuate the bad eating habits that lead to being overweight. Again, the important point is that this answer only puts limits on your motivation to change. Ultimately, you have to ask yourself what body shape you would like to have and how hard you are willing to work at it. If you are five feet three and have seen three generations of roly-poly relatives and have had that general shape yourself since early childhood, you may have to work quite hard to reduce and to keep your weight and shape in the form that is your ideal. While it may be harder for you than for someone else, it's your choice to make. Overweight women often have to face this issue when they see that men seem to have a somewhat easier time losing weight.

As for neurosis being the reason for obesity, it is our judgment that this explanation is a blind alley. Too many people are overweight; some of them are neurotics, but no higher a percentage than in the rest of the population. If you feel that you have serious psychological problems, either related to your weight or not, we recommend that you see a mental health professional. Your physician or local mental health association can give you some referrals if you need them.

Other explanations for obesity heard occasionally include food allergies or compulsive addiction to one food, such as chocolate. While we don't deny that sweets are an important problem for many overweight people, we have rarely, if ever, seen someone whose primary problem is a fatal attraction to one food.

Setting aside the type of broad, general explanations we have been discussing will help you face the fact that being overweight is a matter of your choice and that a commitment to learning the skills of permanent weight control is a difficult but do-able task. There are some other questions about your life and attitude toward being overweight that *do* seem to us to be profitable to ask as you begin a new effort to change. Unlike the general *why* questions, these may provide you with some insights that have practical implications for your effort.

First, how important is being overweight? If you have been noticeably overweight for much of your life, you have had many experiences that contribute to your self-image about body size. Say these adjectives to yourself, and see which ones seem to fit: fat, obese, chubby, plump, tubby, flabby. For most overweight people these words hurt, even if you've never actually heard someone call you one of them. Yet not everyone sees his weight as a liability. You might remember such public figures as Fats Domino, Chubby Checker, Two Ton Tony Galento. Aside from commercial use of the labels, many people who have been overweight for many years see a positive side of the condition. They see being big as being powerful or healthy. They seem to revel in being noticed, even if the attention is negative. I refer to this as the black-sheep syndrome, not unlike the lonely child who acts naughty to get his parents' attention. Your awareness of these possibilities is important because the reactions of people to your weight-loss efforts and your attachment to a body image will affect your motivation as you proceed. If you see slim as weak or fat as being the life of the party, change will be threatening. Your awareness can forearm you and help prevent this attack on your motivation.

The other side of the body image problem is the belief that only slim is beautiful and that all of life's benefits center on being slim. Listen to sentences like, "If only I were slim, I'd have a beautiful wife." "If I were slim, I'd get that promotion." Unrealistic hopes can be as damaging to motivation as holding on to the mythical advantages of being large. As we have indicated, maintenance is as critical as weight loss, in the long run. If you lose weight and don't find yourself receiving all of those expected benefits, the chances of slipping back into old habits are increased. Now is a good time to review your expectations and to include in your commitment to lose weight the understanding that other changes may be necessary to achieve goals that are only partially related to weight.

Another important step in securing the best motivation is the

setting of a weight-loss goal. There are various ways to do this, if you don't already have an ideal weight in mind. There are height-weight tables such as most physicians use to advise patients. Those give you an acceptable range and may be useful if they take into account body frame and age. Your goal might also be stated in terms of body measurements or clothing size. However you set your goal, two principles are important. First, be prepared to change the goal. As you approach a goal you may realize you want to be somewhat above or below the original figure. Settling for a higher weight is a difficult conflict some of you may have to face. On the one hand, not reaching your original goal may leave you psychologically vulnerable to feeling a failure and then regaining the weight you have lost. On the other hand, you may feel quite relieved to face the fact that the cost of maintaining a lower weight is too great and that a slightly higher weight leaves you feeling fit and comfortable. The second principle is that you must have intermediate goals on the way to the final goal. These are points at which you can reward yourself and feel the satisfaction of progress.

Failures are a major threat to motivation. Most of you have tried to lose weight before and have failed. How did you react to that failure? Did you blame the diet, the person helping you, your spouse, events in your life, your own weakness? You will fail again. It may shock you to hear that, but it's a reality that is important to face. No weight-loss effort is perfectly smooth and without failures, which are hopefully temporary but nevertheless discouraging. Your attitude toward failure is an important determinant to long-term motivation. This book does not present a single-minded, unified regime; it's a collection of techniques that you can individually tailor to your needs. When you fail, you should blame the techniques you are using. We want you to take an educational, problem-solving approach. If something isn't working, try something else until you get back on track.

We would like to close this view of the general area of motivation by asking you to review your life situation for obstacles that may get in your way. Are you in the midst of a crisis (marital problems, a job change)? Sometimes such crises can motivate us to change a lot at once—lose weight, quit smoking, learn a new sport, etc. You have to assess whether to address the crisis first or to take on the weight-loss task. We can't give you a formula for the best timing, but we think you can consider the alternatives and safely postpone weight loss if you decide that's best.

While we have said that it is rare for there to be a medical cause of obesity, your health may be an important determinant of your success in weight loss. While it is quite possible to lose weight slowly and safely without medical supervision, if you have any concerns about your health, seeing your physician can be an important step to clear the way for beginning your weight-loss program.

Finally, you might take a look at life roles that play an important part in your weight problem. Working as a cook, feeding a large family, working around food, breastfeeding, inability to exercise, an unusually heavy work schedule—any of these may make weight loss especially difficult. These are situations that may be difficult to change, though you may want to examine the possibilities closely. Awareness of these factors, even if you can't change them, can alert you to strategies that can allow you to succeed even in the face of the obstacle.

Now that we have taken a general look at the problem of motivation, here are several specific exercises that will help you increase your motivation to control your weight.

First, take a sheet of paper and write at the top, "What are my excuses?" Divide the paper with a line down the middle. On the left side list all of the excuses you make for not controlling your eating, for not getting more exercise, for not taking any of the steps you need to take. List them clearly and number them. On the right-hand side, next to each excuse, briefly write a counter-argument to that excuse. Be your own critic and mentally say "Baloney" to each excuse, writing down the reasons why the excuse is not really valid. It may be that some of the problems you list are really serious, but you can always argue that none of them is so tough as to justify hurting yourself even further by overeating. Whatever the situation, if you *feel* stronger you will do better in dealing with it. And you know one thing that controlling your eating does for you—you *feel* stronger, more confident.

A second concrete step you can take to increase your motivation is to make a visual reminder. Take an index card and title it, "My Reasons to Lose Weight." List as many reasons as you can think of. Be very specific about those reasons. For example, instead of saying "To improve my health," list a *specific* improvement that will really be personally meaningful to you, such as "To be less short of breath" or "To reduce my high blood pressure." Put the card somewhere where you will read it at least once a day (just before a meal is an ideal time). Also, carry a copy in your wallet or purse and read it when you are tempted to "mis-eat." This is our word for overeating, short for "mistaken eating." We like the concept of mistaken eating—an honest mistake—rather than the usual idea that you have somehow "cheated."

A third way to increase your motivation is to take an honest look at your own body. This means standing in front of a full-length mirror, in the nude. This is a very difficult assignment for many people. We have the habit of seeing only what we want to see in a mirror—our hair, our face for shaving or putting on makeup, our clothes. Really looking at the body can be quite upsetting. Before you try it, a couple of ground rules are important for you to know. First, it's a good idea to accept the principle expressed by Alcoholics Anonymous and here paraphrased: "Give me the strength to know what I can change and what I can't, and to accept the difference." Losing weight can make you generally smaller, especially along with physical exercise to tighten muscles. Losing weight will probably *not* change your basic proportions. If you tend to be bigger in the hips than in the chest, that difference will persist after you become generally smaller. The second thing to remember in looking in the mirror is that you should focus on your strong points as well as your weak ones. Notice what you like about your appearance even though you're overweight—the shape of your facial features, the texture of your skin, your hair, your nails, your feet and hands, neck, ears—everything counts! Try to imagine how you would like to look; close your eyes and see if you can get that image as clearly as possible. If you have a photograph of yourself when you were slimmer, take a close look at it. We've even had people ask one of those sketch artists you see at fairs or amusement parks to sketch them as they would look if they were slim. Speaking of photos, it can be useful for motivation to have a good picture of yourself now. Post the photos somewhere where you can see them regularly, to be reminded of your goal.

As you lose weight your clothing becomes an important factor in your motivation. Feeling those large sizes get baggy will be very encouraging. You want to get rid of larger-size clothes, except perhaps for one outfit to look at as a reminder. Occasionally, buy an outfit a bit too small as an incentive to lose enough to get into it.

The use of new clothes as an incentive relates to an important general principle: Self-control is not some mysterious power that we are born with. It is an ongoing process with several parts. First, our self-control is determined by our environment. It is a lot harder to avoid temptation if you work in a bakery than if you are a mail carrier. Second, we make decisions or commitments to change strong habits. Repeating these commitments to ourselves (to lose weight, quit smoking) helps us to take the other steps necessary to effect self-control. That's why we suggested looking in the mirror and evaluating your self-labels to help you make the commitment, and making a "Reasons to Lose Weight" list to remind yourself of that commitment. Commitment alone rarely produces change in self-control. You must acquire and make a lot of different self-controlling responses, some of which are directly involved in the goal (e.g., eating less or exercising more), and some of which are less immediate (e.g., changing your environment or learning to be more assertive). The rest of this book can be viewed as training in various self-control skills. An important self-control skill is self-reward. New clothes hanging in a closet serve to remind you of your commitment and to reward you when you carry out the commitment. Generally, we are motivated to do what is rewarding. Change on the scale or with the tape measure is too slow and too erratic to fulfill all of our needs for reward. That's why we emphasize such self-rewards as keeping a list of victories over temptations to read regularly to remind yourself of progress.

We have just referred to *self*-reward as a part of self-control. Most of us have learned to rely heavily on external, social reward to motivate and reinforce our behavior. A verbal pat on the head, or its opposite in the form of criticism, can have dramatic effects on our self-control. There is a balance between relying on self-reward and relying on feedback from others. That balance is a personal one which you should evelute for yourself. On the one hand, you may want to tell certain important people about your weight-control efforts and encourage them to praise you for certain behaviors and for changes in weight. We have worked with people who have even arranged for long-term rewards or punishments from other people for reaching, or not reaching, a weight goal (a vacation, giving money to an unappealing cause for failing to meet a goal, etc.). The effectiveness of this kind of external motivator varies from person to person. You may prefer to keep the whole process to yourself and provide your own rewards.

Another pitfall we have to avoid in thinking about motivation is the "on the wagon—off the wagon" mentality. This is the view that you are either totally good, sticking to your diet, doing all of your assignments, or you are totally bad, off the wagon. Self-control is a variable thing. Your goal should not be perfect control, but an effort to increase the proportion of times when you make the choices in the direction of your overall commitment to control your eating. There will be good days and not-so-good days. What determines this is not always clear—it may be health, quality of sleep, weather, biorhythms, expectations for the coming day, events the day before. But we often seem to sense early in the day how we feel and how the day may go. Is there anything to do other than go back to bed and pull the covers over our heads?

Suppose you wake up feeling kind of blah or even upset or anxious—some low-motivation state. Here are some steps to increase your changes of reversing the tide:

1. Try not to start off the day with yesterday's clouds hanging over you. Obviously, some problems continue, but often we unnecessarily rehash yesterday, being critical of our own and others' behavior. Let go of yesterday as much as you can. Sometimes a simple phrase helps, such as, "Today is (whatever date), a new day in my life."

2. Don't expect yourself to leap in, full steam ahead. Some of us are slow starters. Try to give yourself *time* for an easy start-up. Find a routine that helps you feel refreshed in the morning. This could involve some physical activity, or a relaxation exercise we'll teach

you (with imagining of pleasant scenes), or a shower, or whatever you find pleasurable. In a family discussion, you may have to assert your need for this time in the morning and get help from others to get what you need.

3. If you find yourself getting tense and "speedy," try telling yourself to slow down and take one step at a time. No matter how full your schedule, this slowing down will make you more productive.

4. Plan some simple goals for the day, tasks you know you can get done. Plan rewards for these goals, specific pleasures you can expect throughout the day.

5. Regardless of tasks or rewards, plan at least one pleasant treat for yourself at a specific time toward the middle of the day (a time to read, some shopping, a relaxing bath, a visit with a friend, a walk, an enjoyable phone call, whatever nice thing you can think of).

On the other hand, suppose you wake up feeling super terrific! The important thing is to take advantage of this strength, but not to overdo. Your calorie intake varies from day to day; that's fine, because it's the weekly average that is critical. But, on those especially strong days, take advantage by keeping your eating to a minimum. You probably will feel less hungry, and you can use the opportunity to bank some calories for a rainy day.

This chapter has covered the problem of motivation, including both general issues of emotions and attitudes affecting weight control as well as specific techniques to analyze and reinforce your motivation. In the coming weeks you should read your "Reasons to Lose Weight" card regularly, and be especially aware of obstacles that reduce your motivation. As you proceed with your weight-control efforts you may want to review this chapter whenever you feel your motivation lagging and in need of reexamination.

chapter three
DIETS OR CALORIE COUNTING: WHERE TO BEGIN?

We said in Chapter 1 that diets are okay, as long as you don't believe the hype and you use them in a sensible way. The important thing to remember is that ultimately you have to maintain your weight without staying on a structured diet, and that you should learn the skills to do that as soon as possible.

Miss Piggy (the Muppet), in her *Guide to Life*, suggests that every diet has some tasty foods and some not so good, and that an ideal approach is to combine the best foods from a bunch of different diets. She comes up with a sample that allows you to eat such goodies as ravioli, chocolate cake, and French fries. Actually, Miss Piggy's sample isn't so farfetched. There have been diets that urge you to eat exotic fruits (carbohydrate), others that advise no carbohydrates and unlimited protein (as much steak as you want), and still others that say fats are fine (plenty of butter and cream). Professional dieticians usually recommend what they call isocalorie diets, consisting of a fixed number of calories, with foods selected from across the basic food groups (see the Nutrition section later in this chapter). The Weight Watchers' program (they avoid the word *diet* and the counting of calories) is the best-known example of the balanced diet.

While Miss Piggy is speaking tongue-in-cheek (not a bad way to avoid chewing), you probably could mix and match from several diets, but only if you stuck to any given diet for several days. Most of the diets you've heard of are not dangerous, if you don't stay on the more extreme ones for more than a week or two. Whether any of them have any special magic is doubtful.

We suggest that if you find structured diets work well for you for a given period of time, choose one or two of your favorites and use them in the way we outline below. If you're concerned about the healthfulness of popular diets, by all means consult your physician or a professional dietician.

Once you've selected a diet and feel ready to begin, go for it! If you stick to most diets for a few days, you will see a loss of several pounds. Most of that will be what's referred to as fluid or water loss, especially if your diet involves a reduction of carbohydrates and fats. You'll feel virtuous and reassured that you're well on your way to your goal. Unfortunately, two negative things begin to happen, sometimes after a few days, sometimes a week or two later (if you're lucky): The weight loss gets smaller and the food on the diet gets very boring. In the end it seems that calories do count and that you will lose only an amount of weight very closely related to the number of calories you've cut out. We've reproduced here a whimsical diet that came to us without reference to source; it cuts out a lot of calories. You can try the Miss Piggy approach and switch diets. The food will be more interesting, we hope, but you probably won't get that initially larger loss you experienced with the first diet.

The Guaranteed Weight-Loss Diet—or your money back

Monday	Breakfast	weak tea
	Lunch	one bouillon cube in one-half cup diluted water
	Dinner	one pigeon thigh, three ounces prune juice (gargle only)
Tuesday	Breakfast	scraped crumbs from burnt toast
	Lunch	one doughnut hole (without sugar), one glass of dehydrated water
	Dinner	three grains of cornmeal, broiled
Wednesday	Breakfast	shredded eggshell skin
	Lunch	one-half dozen poppy seeds
	Dinner	bee's knees and mosquito knuckles, sautéed in vinegar

Thursday	Breakfast	boiled-out stains of old tablecloth
	Lunch	belly button of a navel orange
	Dinner	three eyes from an Irish potato, diced
Friday	Breakfast	two lobster antennas
	Lunch	one tail joint of sea horse
	Dinner	rotisserie-broiled guppy fillet
Saturday	Breakfast	four chopped banana seeds
	Lunch	broiled butterfly liver
	Dinner	jelly vertebra of la centipede
Sunday	Breakfast	pickled hummingbird tongue
	Lunch	prime rib of tadpole, aroma of empty custard pie plate
	Dinner	tossed paprika and clover leaf salad

NOTE: A seven-ounce glass of steam may be consumed on alternate days to help in having something to blow off.

So, what's the answer? It's simple; perhaps discouraging in the short run, but has excellent prospects for the long run. Intentionally go off the diet. Don't feel guilty. Put it away in a drawer with the full knowledge that you will use it again—and again, and again—but when you need it or want it. The choice and the control are yours. When you decide to drop somebody else's diet, you'll begin to select foods from your own normal diet. The trick, of course, is to control *how much you eat*, not which foods you eat. To do that, you'll need a guide to control quantity. That means knowing portion size and counting calories.

We can picture you throwing up your hands in disgust at this point and saying something like, "Oh no, not me; I'm not going to carry around a calorie book and an adding machine for the rest of my life."

If you've picked us up off the floor and are plowing ahead again, please be assured that it is not our intention to tie you to a complicated calorie-counting system. On the contrary, we will be showing you how to simplify calorie knowledge and record keeping. Within a short time you'll be able to keep a simple record without referring to books or weighing your food. A brief period of learning will give you tremendous flexibility in your selection of food, not only while you're losing weight but, more importantly, when you're maintaining your weight—for the rest of your life. You'll be able to use a natural selection of your own favorite foods, controlling quantity and allowing you to lose weight at a good, safe pace. Then, when you want to or when you feel the need, you can pull out your favorite diet for a few days and use it with confidence. You can even shift over to this system gradually; for example, starting with calorie counting one day a week, then two days, and so on. Later in this chapter we'll show you in detail how to do this.

Before presenting a brief summary of nutrition principles, we would like to say a bit about fasting. In the next chapter we suggest that you learn about hunger by trying a brief fast (one day) if you've never had that experience. That suggestion is not made as a method of weight loss. Fasting has a long and controversial history. It has been used for religious enlightenment, for alleged body purification, and for drastic weight loss. Complete fasting (water or noncalorie liquids only) can be dangerous after a couple of days. Most people will have no serious negative effects, but some will. So we recommend that you never fast completely without medical supervision. If a medical person, or any other professional, urges you to fast completely for more than a week, we urge you to get a second opinion.

By now most dieters have heard of protein liquid (or powder) fasting, sometimes referred to as a *protein-sparing fast*. One of the negative effects of complete fasting is that your body cannot fully distinguish between fat and muscle. After a while on a complete fast you begin to lose weight not only by burning up your stores of extra fat but also by burning muscle tissue—clearly not a desirable result. In theory, eating a small amount of protein-bearing food every day prevents the loss of body muscle. Whether or not the theory proves valid, it is clear that many people have lost a lot of weight relatively quickly using this system *under a physician's direction*. The problem remains: What do you do when the fasting period is over? You could simply go back on the fast if you regained weight, but that seems to lead to an ultimately ineffective and perhaps damaging yo-yo syndrome. Physicians specializing in the fasting approach are increasingly recognizing that permanent weight loss requires the patients' learning what leads them to overeat and how to control eating when the fast ends.

So, you're right back where you started. In essence, there is no escaping the type of learning presented in this book. You might as well begin now, whether you decide to diet or fast just for a while, or even all the way to your goal. You will have the best chance for maintenance if you accept the need for this learning and begin it now. If you wait until you reach your goal weight, there is a serious danger that you will say, in effect, "I'm cured; I don't have to bother with learning about calorie counting, increasing physical activity, or the psychology of overeating." That would be a serious error and would likely result in your becoming another statistic in the depressingly large number of people who regain all of the weight they've lost.

After the nutrition review, the rest of this chapter shows you how to keep a simple diary of your eating, weight, physical activity, and the factors contributing to your loss of eating control. Whether or not you are planning to use a diet or fast for a while, make the effort now to get the diary habit and to go on to establish your own system of self-control, using the methods suggested in the remainder of the book.

NUTRITION

While this book focuses mostly on the psychological issues related to weight reduction and control, we would like to give you a few general pointers about what you eat. This is only a very brief, traditional introduction to accepted principles of nutrition.

Basic Food Groups

There are four basic food groups. You should select as wide a variety of foods as you can from the four groups.

1. Milk—including cheese and ice cream.
2. Meat—including fish, poultry, and eggs. Dry beans (such as soya), dry peas, and nuts also substitute for meat products.
3. Vegetables and fruits—include some citrus (orange, grapefruit, tangerine), some green leafy, as well as yellow or root vegetables.
4. Bread and cereal—including grits, noodles, rice, and macaroni or spaghetti.

Basic Nutrients Contained
in Various Foods

CARBOHYDRATES. Carbohydrates are the most important source of the energy you need for all your daily activities. Important sources of carbohydrates are whole-grain cereals and breads, potatoes, dried fruits, and bananas. Although much maligned by dieters, they are essential suppliers of energy most readily available for use by the body.

PROTEIN. Protein is the fundamental structural element of every body cell. Proteins build and repair body tissues, help fight infection, and serve as a source of food energy. Best sources of protein are meat, poultry, fish, eggs, milk, cheese, soybeans, nuts, and dry beans and peas.

FATS. Fats play several roles in the body. They are a primary source of energy and body warmth. Certain kinds of fats furnish vitamin A or D; some fish-liver oils, for example, provide both. Moreover, fats help the body make use of these vitamins, helping to absorb them in the intestinal tract.

There is a controversy among nutritionists about the value of a low-carbohydrate diet for reducing. Generally, our philosophy is that a balanced intake is best since it is most similar to the food program you will live with for the rest of your life. *Any radical diet should be used only as a means of getting going in your weight reduction, with a shift back to a balanced intake before or when you reach your goal weight.* In this way, you learn self-control while eating all of your familiar foods.

Even within a balanced diet, however, you should know that the three types of nutrients vary in the number of calories they contain. Fats are very high in calories (about nine per gram), carbohydrates and proteins relatively lower (about five per gram). Therefore, you can reduce your total calorie intake most easily by reducing amounts of fat. Trim away all excess fat from meats; minimize fat in cooking (use nonstick pans and shift away from frying whenever possible while still keeping your meals tasty). minimize butter and margarine on breads (get the taste you want from a "scraping" of butter rather than a thick layer). It is probably better to get your fats in vegetable form (for example, corn oil) rather than from meat or dairy products, to keep cholesterol intake down. Your doctor can tell you if this should be a special concern for you. Try to get your sugar naturally in fruits, rather than in sugary desserts. Avoid adding sugar; use saccharine or other low-calorie substitutes. Use diet food substitutes *if* you like the taste; especially try the low-calorie soft drinks if you like this type of drink.

VITAMINS AND MINERALS.   If you eat a reasonably balanced diet, you should get enough of these. If your doctor recommends it, or if you would feel more comfortable, consider taking a multivitamin tablet.

LIQUIDS.   Drink plenty of low-calorie fluids, especially water. Drinking a liquid just before a meal may help reduce hunger. During meals, drink between bites, when your mouth is clear of food. Do not wash away the taste of food by drinking with food in your mouth.

SALT.   It is probably best to keep your salt intake from being excessive. Explore other seasonings. This may be a special problem for some overweight people who retain body fluids or suffer from high blood pressure. Check with your physician if you have any concerns about this.

ROUGHAGE OR BULK.   Your diet should contain enough whole-grain foods (for example, bran and uncooked vegetables and fruit) to keep your bowels moving regularly. Again, consult your physician if you have problems in this regard.

MEAL PATTERN.   Generally, the adage "Eat a good breakfast" is a useful one. However, *some* overweight people can be very successful by skipping breakfast. We urge you to experiment with this for yourself. You can balance your diet without breakfast. You may need some juice, if nothing else, to keep you from feeling light-headed. You can also experiment with the number and spacing of other meals. Some people do better on three meals, some on four or five smaller meals. Some do better with only a light meal in the evening. You must find your own best way.

There are many other nutritional issues that are beyond the scope of this book. We recommend that you check with your physician or other resource person, or test out the effects of variations in diet content for yourself.

The remainder of this chapter orients you to a basic tool of this program—the diary. Whether or not you are ready to begin to control food intake with calorie counting, we recommend that you begin to learn how to do so. You may decide to use only parts of the diary now—for example, recording your exercise and noticing the times you snack and the emotions that lead you to overeat. Then you'll be ready to use the diary fully when you decide to begin the switch from dieting to calorie counting.

The first page of the diary is divided into three sections: food intake with the number of calories, amount of extra physical activity (how many minutes and how many calories this activity burned up), and *how much you weigh*. The three divisions are labeled food diary, extra physical activity diary, and weight diary.

This diary will show you your energy balance. Each person has his own unique body machine. Fuel is taken in as potential energy. This fuel is burned up by physical activity as well as being used to keep your body temperature constant, and to keep your internal functions operating. When there is excess fuel for these purposes, it gets converted to fat and stored for future use. On the other hand, if on any given day you do not take in enough fuel, your body machinery draws on its storage, burning up fat (and, of course, lowering your weight). Although your machine may not be perfectly predictable each day, over the days you will begin to see the expected pattern.

For the first week that you use the Food Diary, you will not have a "daily caloric goal" (see upper right-hand corner of the diary). Instead, we want you to observe your current eating habits, whatever your diet is. Don't attempt a stringent cut in calories, but also try not to use this week as an excuse for "one last binge." You will have a picture at the end of the week of where you are *now* in your eating habits and energy balance.

The Food Diary is a day-by-day account of *everything* you eat.

Name _____ Week Beginning _____ Daily Calorie Goal _____

My Average for this Week _____

FOOD DIARY

Monday		Tuesday		Wednesday		Thursday		Friday		Saturday		Sunday	
Foods	Cal.	Foods	Cal.	Foods	Cal.	Foods	Cal.	Foods	Cal.	Foods	Cal.	Foods	Cal.
Total		Total		Total		Total		Total		Total		Total	

EXTRA PHYSICAL ACTIVITY DIARY

Monday		Tuesday		Wednesday		Thursday		Friday		Saturday		Sunday	
Minutes	Cal.	Minutes	Cal.	Minutes	Cal.	Minutes	Cal.	Minutes	Cal.	Minutes	Cal.	Minutes	Cal.
Total		Total		Total		Total		Total		Total		Total	

WEIGHT DIARY

Monday	Tuesday	Wednesday	Thursday	Friday	Saturday	Sunday	Mon. A.M.

FOOD	TYPICAL SERVING	CALORIES	
BEVERAGES			
Beer	12-ounce can	150	
Cocktails, Highballs	3-ounce glass	200	
Cola and other nondiet soda	8-ounce glass	100	
Hot Chocolate	6-ounce cup	160	
Ice Cream Soda	Fountain serving	500	
Juices: Grape or Prune	4-ounce glass	90	
Other Fruit		50	
Lemonade	8-ounce glass	100	
Malted Milk or Milkshake	Fountain Serving	700	
Milk: Whole	8-ounce glass	160	
Low Fat		120	
Nonfat Milk, Buttermilk		80	
Wine: Dry	4-ounce glass	100	
Sweet		140	
DAIRY			
Butter (also Margarine, oil)	1 Tablespoon	100	Pat 70
Cheese	1-ounce slice	100	1-inch cube 120
Cottage Cheese	1/2 cup	100	
Cream Cheese	1 Tablespoon	60	
Coffee Cream	1 Tablespoon	30	
Whipped Cream	1 Tablespoon, level	35	
Yogurt (flavored)	8-ounce cup	240	
Sour Cream	1 Tablespoon	25	
EGGS			
Scrambled or Fried	Each	125	
Other Styles	Each	100	
FISH			
Broiled or Boiled Fish	4 ounces	100	
Fried Fish	4 ounces	300	
Lobster (whole), Broiled	1 pound	120	
Sardines (drained), Salmon (drained)	3-ounce can	200	

28

Food	Serving	Calories	Serving	Calories
Shrimp: Boiled	4 ounces	100		
Batter Fried	4 ounces	300		
Tuna (drained) canned	3-ounce can	200		

FLOUR FOODS

Food	Serving	Calories	Serving	Calories
Bread	1 slice	60	1/2 slice	30
Bagels, Biscuits, Rolls, Muffins	Each	150	half	75
Cereal: Cooked	8-ounce cup	150		
Dry, cold		130		
Crackers	Each	20		
French Toast	Slice	150		
Pancakes	Each, 4" diameter	60		
Pasta: Noodles, Macaroni, Spaghetti	8-ounce cup	200		
With Sauce or Cheese	8-ounce cup	400		
Pizza	1 slice (small)	250		
Tortillas	Each	50		
Waffle	4" x 5"	200		

FRUIT

Food	Serving	Calories	Serving	Calories
Apples (and other round fruit)	1 medium	70	quarter	20
Avocado	1/2 medium	200		
Bananas	1 medium	90	half	45
Cantaloupe	1/2 cup	100		
Canned Fruit With Syrup	1/2 of a 5-inch-long Melon	40	quarter	20
Cherries (fresh)	8-ounce cup	80	each	4
Dates, Figs (small, fresh)	Each	30		
Fresh Fruit Cup	3/4 cup	90		
Grapes	3" x 3" bunch	50		
Grapefruit	1/2 medium	50		
Olives	Each	10		
Pears	Medium, each	100		
Pineapple (fresh)	1/2 cup	40		
Prunes (dried)	Each	20		
Raisins	1 Tablespoon	30		
Strawberries: Fresh	8-ounce cup	50	each (average size)	4
Frozen	3-ounce package	90		

Tomatoes Fresh	1 medium	30		
Canned or Stewed	8-ounce cup	50		
Watermelon	1-inch thick, slice	60		

MEAT AND FOWL

Bacon	Medium slice	50		
Beef or Veal (cooked)	4-ounce portion	300		
Beef Liver (broiled)	4-ounce portion	200		
Beef, ground (cooked)	1/4 pound (4 ounces)	350		
Other (Pork, Lamb, Ham)	4-ounce portion	400		
Lunch Meat (Bologna, etc.)	1-ounce slice	100		
Hot Dog (without roll)	1 average	130		
Chicken: Broiled or Boiled	4 ounces	150		
Roasted	4 ounces	200		
Pan Fried	4 ounces	250		
Batter-Deep-Fried with Skin	4 ounces	300		
Duck	4 ounces	250		
Turkey (Roasted)	4 ounces	300		

SALADS (includes 1 Tablespoon of mayonnaise)

Chicken Salad	1 cup (including 1 Tbsp. mayo)	250	1/2 cup	125
Cole Slaw	2/3 cup (dressed)	100		
Potato Salad	1/2 cup (incl. 1 Tbsp. mayo)	200		
Salmon Salad	1 cup (including 1 Tbsp. mayo)	500	1/2 cup	250
Shrimp Salad	1 cup (including 1 Tbsp. mayo)	300	1/2 cup	150
Tuna Salad (drained canned tuna)	1 cup (including 1 Tbsp. mayo)	400	1/2 cup	200
Tossed, Mixed Salad	1 cup (without dressing)	40		

SANDWICHES

(includes the calories for bread with mayonnaise or butter plus calories for filling)

Hamburger	1 quarter-pound patty	600	1/2 sandwich	300
Cheeseburger	1 quarter-pound patty	700	1/2 sandwich	350
Low-Calorie Sandwiches: Lettuce and Tomato, Chicken, Fish, Eggs, Hot Dog, Bacon	average thickness	300		
Medium-Calorie Sandwiches:				

Item	Measure	Calories		
Chopped liver, roast beef, corned beef, pastrami, chicken salad	average thickness	400		
High-Calorie Sandwiches:				
Ham, Cheese, Turkey, Tuna Salad, Salami	average thickness	500		
Tacos	each	350		
SAUCES, DRESSINGS, GRAVIES				
Creamy, Mayonnaise	1 Tablespoon	100	1 teaspoon	35
Others (including medium-thick gravy)	1 Tablespoon	50	1 teaspoon	20
Ketchup, Mustard, Relish	1 Tablespoon	30	1 teaspoon	10
SOUPS				
Clear Broth	8-ounce cup	50		
Creamed Soups	8-ounce cup	200		
Others	8-ounce cup	100		
SWEETS AND SNACKS				
Cakes: Cheesecake	Average Wedge	300		
Chocolate Layer Cake, Iced	Average Wedge	400		
Cupcake	Each	200		
Doughnut (Iced or Sugared)	Each	200		
Brownie	Average Piece	200		
Cookies	Each	60		
Candy: Chocolate	Small Bar	150		
Fancy Chocolates	1/4 lb.	500	1 piece	100
Hard	1 Piece	25		
Honey	1 teaspoon	20		
Ice Cream: Banana Split	Fountain size	1500		
Chocolate Sundae	1 scoop	500		
Cone	1 scoop	350		
Dish	1 scoop	300		
Jam	1 teaspoon	20		
Jell-o, plain	8-ounce cup	150		
Nuts (including peanut butter)	1 Tablespoon (8-12 nuts)	100		
Pastry	1 medium piece	250		
Pie	1 average slice	300		

		Calories		
Popcorn (plain, no butter)	small box	100		
Crackerjacks	1-ounce box	120		
Potato Chips	small bag (1 oz.)	150	each potato chip	10
Pretzels (3-ring)	small bag	200	each pretzel	10
Pudding or Custard	1/2 cup	150		
Sherbet	1/2 cup	120		
Sugar	1 Tablespoon	60	1 teaspoon	20
Syrup	1 Tablespoon	60	1 teaspoon	20

VEGETABLES

*Group 1: High-Calorie Vegetables

Beans, Baked	1 cup	300		
Corn on the cob	1 ear, 6 inches	100		
Chili	1 cup	400		
Chop Suey	1 cup	300		
Hominy	1 cup	120		
Potatoes: Baked or Boiled	1 medium	100		
French Fried	1 serving	200	each French fry	20
Mashed (with milk and butter)	1 cup	200		
Sweet (candied)	2 halves	300	1 half	150
Rice, boiled	1 cup	200		

**Group 2: Medium-Calorie Vegetables

	1 cup	100	

Artichokes, Beans, Beets, Corn (canned), Peas, Pumpkin, Rutabaga, Winter Squash

***Group 3: Low-Calorie Vegetables

	1 cup	50	

Spinach, Mushrooms, Celery, Lettuce, Cabbage, Cucumber, Raw Onions, Carrots, Broccoli, Cauliflower, Turnips

DIARY NOTES

Include the situations or the feelings that made you overeat
  (example of a situation: argument with husband, pressure at work, mother's criticism)
  (example of a feeling: felt frustrated, or bored, or angry, or sad, or sexual, or tense, etc.)
Include your victories and star them. (example: *resisted offer of candy at the office)

Monday	Tuesday	Wednesday	Thursday
Friday	Saturday	Sunday	In General (persistent things)

How to figure how many calories you are burning up:

Light Activity: 3 Calories Per Minute	Medium Activity: 5 Calories Per Minute	Heavy: 7 Per Minute
walking, bicycling, gardening	swimming, fast walking, rowing	tennis, skiing, running, handball

33

We emphasize *everything* because it is crucial that you take complete responsibility for your eating. This is your record. It is your way of keeping track and of learning to be honest with yourself. The first time you mis-eat or even binge you will be tempted not to write it down or to change the calories. Don't cheat yourself. The only way you'll learn from your mistakes is by seeing them recorded. The diary is compact so that you can photocopy it and carry it around with you at all times. It's small, so you will have to write small.

In the column marked Food, abbreviate the name of each food you eat; record the number of calories in the next column. Also, note the time of day you ate your meal or snack, so that you can review your diary to learn when you danger times are. Record your eating as soon as possible; memory quickly fades.

In order to simplify the record keeping, the Simplified Calorie Chart we've given you in the diary deliberately has the numbers rounded off to the nearest ten and takes averages for many foods (for example, all cookies are called sixty calories). It's more important that you be consistent than exact with your number records. Calorie books often disagree with each other. Your purpose is to have a picture of how much you are eating. Then you will know how much to cut down in order to lose weight.

Our chart naturally omits many foods. To include them all would defeat our whole purpose in inventing a *simplified* calorie counter. We are not interested in having you tote a heavy calorie counter around with you. When you eat a food and find it is not on our chart, we urge you to make an educated guess, based on the items that *are* listed. If you would like, you can consult your favorite book of calorie values; most book stores carry several. We left a few blank lines for you to write in additions that you *frequently* eat. Gradually, you must begin memorizing how many calories are in the foods you eat, so that you have condensed our already-condensed chart even further! Don't get hooked on a calorie-counting book. By gradually memorizing a relatively short list (probably about one hundred foods), you will be able to monitor yourself easily and gain the freedom to make knowledgeable choices.

All calorie values are for single foods, unless specified (waffles *without* any topping). For casseroles, you'll have to figure by combining contents, unless they consist of one predominant food (like beef). For dietetic foods, use the calorie value on the package. If none is given, use the value for a nondietetic version.

The Calories column of your diary will contain the calorie value for *each* food you eat. For example, if you ate two slices of toast, each with a pat of butter, the total calories to record would be 220 (60 for each slice of bread, 50 for each pat of butter). Keep subtotals of your calories frequently as you go through the day, so you will know where you stand. This will be particularly useful to you when you have a daily calorie goal you are aiming for.

Gradually, you will begin to see your diary as a bank account. You'll be able to see where you can save calories and when you have saved a nest egg of calories, perhaps to be spent on a rainy day or on some upcoming happy occasion. You'll also know if you're running in the red, and how much you have to cut back to balance the account, either for that day or for a several-day period.

Actually measure and weigh your food for the first two weeks. Gradually, you will learn to judge by eye, so that you won't have to depend on a scale or measuring cup. As you record, you will be learning calorie values. In a few weeks you'll know from memory the value of the foods you eat most frequently.

At the end of the first seven days, find out what your average is by adding up all the daily calorie totals and dividing by seven. Put the average in the space in the upper right-hand corner of the Food Diary, marked My Average for this Week.

Let us now look at the Extra Physical Activity part of the diary just below. Most of us only use the word *calories* when we talk about how much food we take in. Actually, calories are a measure of energy—energy potential in food and energy burned by your body. When we do any physical activity, we are burning up calories that we took into the body by eating.

The Extra Physical Activity Diary is to record *extra* calories above those expended in your normal daily activity. The purpose is to give you a guide to output so that you can gradually increase it and produce both a better weight loss and a new pattern of more activity that will help keep the weight off. Therefore, only record physical exercise or extra activity *above your usual level.* (You don't subtract these calories from your food calories in your diary).

You see by referring to the list printed on your diary that different activities or exercise burn calories at different rates. For example, bicycling burns up three calories per minute, while playing tennis burns up seven calories per minute. The exact rates are determined by many factors: your weight, speed of movements, the air temperature, etc. As a rule of thumb—to give you a guide— if you huff and puff in ten minutes, call it *heavy* exercise (seven extra calories per minute); if you huff and puff in a half hour, call it *moderate exercise* (five calories per minute); if you can go on for an hour or more with no heavy breathing, call it *light* exercise (three calories per minute).

You can see that you can burn up just as many calories walking as running; it just takes longer. You can use this record to plan an exercise program for yourself, or as a tool to offset heavy eating days. You don't have to deduct exercise calories from your daily intake calories; view them as a bonus to each day's efforts.

The third diary section is the weight diary. Weigh yourself daily, at the same time and in the same state of dress. It may be painful at first and sometimes discouraging. But it is another important part of commitment and honesty with yourself. If you don't weigh, you know you're hiding and need corrective action. Soon your scale will become your friend, not your enemy; and that daily knowledge will be a vital part of a lifetime of self-control.

On the last sheet of the diary is a place for Diary Notes. Use this each day to note any observations about yourself, but particularly two types of experience:

1. Overeating events, either at meals or snacks. Note the time, situation (especially persons or stressful experiences), and any emotion you experience prior to or during the eating.

2. Victories. Note times you resisted temptation and how you felt. You can also record any other observations about your eating or other aspects of your life. This diary is private. Use it to say anything. Even the first week of the diary will show you a great deal about yourself that will be useful when you begin to explore the problem areas discussed in the rest of the book. You can save the diaries and reread them. Review your diary at the end

of each week. Notice bad times and good times. Notice how your food intake affected the scale the next day. Notice how a day with a lot of exercise may have changed the picture. Your goal is to be learning and always becoming more aware of your own body's energy system and your own pattern of eating problems.

Occasionally we hear someone say, "My only problem is that I love food." Most people strike a balance between eating to live and living to eat. Your defining yourself as overweight and wanting to change means that you are not satisfied with that balance. You have to go beyond the statement "I love food." Self-control consists of commitment to change, awareness of your own behavior patterns, and skills to bring about the change. Your diary, in addition to helping you monitor calories and energy balance, provides you with a major tool for self-awareness. As you write in your diary, you will begin to see patterns in your eating, your activity, and other aspects of your life that contribute to your weight problems. Looking for these patterns may be difficult, but it is essential to get you to face the task of change and to succeed.

There are many theories about food, exercise, weight, appetite, emotional causes of overeating—about every aspect of the weight problem. You can hardly pick up a popular magazine or newspaper without seeing a report of a new theory or a piece of research that promises the solution to all of the problems. Our experience indicates that the best advice we can give people is to do your own research. You are your own best subject. You should constantly be experimenting with every aspect of your eating, physical activity, and other related psychological factors. Accept no recommendations blindly, including those in this book. Test them out, and use your diary as your scientific data sheet, recording the results in your eating, activity, mood, and sense of self-control. This flexible, experimenting orientation will, in the long run, allow you to build a personal control system uniquely tailored to your needs, a system that can change as you change.

Here are a few examples of theories you can test out for yourself in the coming weeks.

Most dieticians recommend that we eat three balanced meals a day and never skip breakfast. Others recommend not eating after

7 P.M. Others say to eat the biggest meal at midday. Should you skip breakfast? What if you are a person who says "If I eat in the morning it makes me hungry—I eat more all day long?" Should you make supper your lightest meal? Test out these theories on yourself. No two people are alike. Build a strategy that works for you. Try eating six small meals a day; try eating your big meal at noon; skip breakfast if you want to. The important thing is to try these ideas one at a time and to systematically record the effects in your diary. Be honest with yourself. If skipping breakfast led you to eat huge lunches, accept the fact that for you, eating breakfast is a good idea, even if it takes a while to get comfortable with that pattern. Or if skipping breakfast turns out to be a good way to save calories, go with *that* idea.

For one week, keep a diary of your food intake, exercise output, and weight, day by day. Even if you have decided to use a structured diet for a while, try recording a diary for a week. Then when you begin using calorie counting regularly, review this chapter and begin to use the calorie part of the diary.

There is another record form on page 203 that you can begin to use whether you're on a diet or calorie counting (or both). It's called the Week-to-Week Record; it consists of three parts: your Sunday weight, your average daily calorie intake that week, and your body masurements, taken once every four weeks.

Weight fluctuates from day to day. As we indicated, we want you to weigh daily. However, for a long-term record the once-a-week weigh-in will give you a more stable picture. You may want to convert these figures to a graph form so that you can see the weight decline more dramatically. Body measurements are a helpful supplementary reinforcement for your efforts. Sometimes you reach a weight plateau, but continuing on your calorie intake level and expending extra physical activity will produce continuing size changes.

Averaging daily calorie intake for a whole week will help you to plan a daily calorie goal for the following week, when you are using calorie counting to control your weight.

When you have recorded in your diary for one week, you will be ready to map out a plan. If you are on a structured diet, we suggest that you still complete a diary form each week, using all of the parts except the calorie section. This will provide you with a great deal of information about your eating patterns and problems and will also help you to structure and control your eating. Then, when you're ready to switch to calorie counting, you can use the calorie column and calculate a calorie goal in the way we are about to describe.

Now, here's the procedure for setting a calorie intake goal.

Compare your *average* calorie intake with your weight. Have you gained, lost, or stayed the same this week?

When you are using calorie counting rather than a structured diet, we want you to lose one to two pounds per week. If you lost in that range this week, then your calorie goal for next week will be the same as your daily calorie average for this week. If your weight stayed the same this week, figure that in order to lose one to two pounds in the coming week, you will have to take in 800 calories *less* each day than you have been doing. So, your daily calorie intake goal will be your present intake minus 800. For example, suppose that the first week you averaged 2300 calories per day and neither lost nor gained any weight. This means that beginning the following week your daily calorie goal should be 1500 calories. Or, if you averaged 2000 and stayed the same, you should try 1200 calories. If you *gained* weight this week, you know you will have to cut down even more than 800 calories per day to start losing weight. This formula will not fit everyone (metabolism and other factors affect the computation), so the following should be your guide for the coming week if you have any doubt about what your goal should be:

Men	1500 calories
Women weighing over 200 pounds	1500 calories
Women weighing 130–200 pounds	1200 calories
Women weighing under 130 pounds	1000 calories

Don't go below 1000 calories for now. If you are one of those rare exceptions who does not lose weight even at 1000 calories, you may want to consult a physician or nutritionist for help. It will take a couple of weeks at a particular calorie level to see how it's working for you. Later, you can adjust your goal up or down to achieve a gradual 1–2 pound loss per week. In the first week with any reduced intake your loss will be higher, so don't be disappointed if your loss is smaller the second week. There also will be periods, for most people, when your calorie intake level no longer seems to be working; you're on a weight loss plateau. Aside from a slight lowering of your calorie goal or increase in your activity, you can try shifting temporarily to a structured diet. Sometimes a sharp reduction in carbohydrates for a few days will get you off the plateau. You may also be retaining fluid and might be helped by medication; again, check with your physician.

Note: *If your current intake is very high (average over 3000 calories), try reducing your intake gradually. Take off 500 calories for a couple of days, then another 500, and so on until you reach a level where you begin to lose weight steadily.*

The goal of a calorie counting system is complete freedom to eat any foods, as long as you monitor the quantity of your intake in a way that will allow you to decrease (or maintain) your weight. This means that your average daily calorie intake for a week should relate fairly closely to your weight change over the week, though daily weight and calorie intake may fluctuate.

The simplified calorie counter allows you to keep track without referring to a complicated book. But eventually we want you to go one step further and learn to be completely independent of any printed calorie counter. Most people regularly eat a fairly limited number of foods; it will be easy to learn the calorie values of this short list of foods.

Each week we want you to try to learn the calories contained in ten to fifteen foods. You can use flash cards and even get a relative or friend to quiz you. Start with the foods you eat most frequently. Keep track of the ones you've learned by marking them off on a photocopy of the calorie chart.

It's also important to learn to judge the quantity of a food by eye. At first you should measure out a quantity of the food, but later you can begin to test your judgment. For example, see how many spoonfuls of a vegetable equals a half-cup portion. How large is a four-ounce hamburger? A few foods require actual weights. You can buy an inexpensive postage scale to help learn to judge this, or you can use premeasured weights from the store. For example, buy a five-ounce piece of beef and cook it; the resulting cooked meat will be fairly close to four ounces. Each week, as you learn the calorie values of foods, practice judging the quantity of those foods by eye or with a common utensil. You can even use your fingers as a ruler. If you know that your forefinger is about four inches long, you can quickly estimate the size of a piece of food in front of you and convert that to weight and calories.

ARE YOU READY TO BEGIN?

When you've reached this point in the book, you have been shown the basic tools to begin not only a weight-loss program, but a complete revamping of your life-style. You must make a choice at this point. You can postpone doing anything and continue your reading. We suggest that you begin now to keep a diary, even if you're uncertain about diets, calorie counting, or even about whether to try to lose weight. That commitment to observe and record will be an important first step. But, you may not be ready to take a first step (actually, you did take the first step when you started reading this). Diets proverbially begin tomorrow, or Monday morning. Don't be hard on yourself for not being ready. You will be in your own good time. You'll wake up one morning feeling especially determined, and you'll be on your way. In the meantime, sit back, relax, and read on. Who knows, an idea in the next chapter may be just the nudge you need.

WORKING WITH A PARTNER

Many of our clients have been married or living with someone; that spouse or friend may or may not have been overweight. Where it was feasible, we found that gaining the cooperation of that person contributed significantly to the progress of the client. Whether you plan to go through this book systematically, week by week, learning the techniques suggested, or you prefer reading for general knowledge and inspiration, you might consider enlisting someone to be your partner during your weight-loss program. This person could also be losing weight, but not in competition with you; or he/she could simply be willing to help you. If you would like to try this partner approach, we suggest that you take three steps:

1. Read Chapter 14 next; hold the family conference suggested there. We have included a Letter to Your Partner at the end of Chapter 14 to introduce your partner (he/she need not be a spouse, of course) to some of the issues involved in helping you. A good way to start the family conference and engage your partner's help would be to have him or her read the letter.

2. Get your partner to read as much of the book as possible as you go along, beginning with the next section.

3. For some chapters we have included a final segment directed to partners, suggesting specific ways to help with the problems and techniques covered in that chapter. Have your partner read a given chapter as you begin to practice the principles and techniques in that chapter, then discuss his/her trying the Suggested Partner Activity at the end.

INTRODUCTION TO A HELPING PARTNER

Having a partner involved in a weight-control program is an important addition to behavioral approaches to weight control. If your partner's past attempts to lose weight have been unsuccessful, or if successes have been temporary, you may have become pessimistic. For this reason we feel it is especially important that you become involved in this new program. There is research showing that a partner can have a powerful impact on eating behavior. Your partner's weight loss may be important to you because of the effects on health, length of life, emotional well-being, and attractiveness. This program is intended to provide you with some ways in which you can be effective in helping him or her stick with this new effort.

We focus on several themes in this book. It is important for you to be aware of what your partner is trying to do. Therefore, it is vital that you read and discuss Chapter 14 and then read any chapter he/she is currently emphasizing. In reading the materials, you may find that the emphasis on changing eating habits—which is a process that takes time—is different from the conventional idea that weight loss is a simple matter of eating less. In order to permanently change eating habits, specific self-control skills must be mastered. By being aware of what your partner is working on, you can know what behavior to encourage and you can gain insight into the amount of effort it takes. After you both read a chapter, discuss the content and decide on several ways you can help carry out some activity for that week.

One general point is important for you to remember: Avoid criticism and nagging as much as possible during the program. Look for changes in behavior related to this program that you can praise or otherwise reward.

We want you to know that we realize that you too are making an important commitment by agreeing to participate. Just as we are asking you to praise your partner's efforts, she (he) should actively guide your help, saying what she (he)* would like you to do and praising you frequently for your efforts. This is to be a mutual project, with work and benefits for you both.

You should be helping out but not trying to do too much or take control. Striking this balance is a delicate matter and will take frank discussions between you. We hope that you will find this not only helpful for your partner's weight problem, but also generally instructive and valuable for you both.

SUGGESTED PARTNER ACTIVITY

This week your partner is beginning to use the Food, Extra Physical Activity, and Weight Diaries to get a picture of body *energy balance*. We suggest that you also keep a diary for *this week only*. Record

*In order to simplify the text, from now on we will use the feminine pronouns *she* and *her* to refer to the program participant, the person working on her weight. For those of you who are partners of male participants, we hope you will bear with us. All of this material is equally applicable regardless of sex. We want only to make the reading of it less cumbersome.

everything you eat, your physical activity, and your weight. Figure your calorie totals at the end of the day with your partner's help. It is important for you to experience keeping a diary so that you can appreciate the amount of effort your partner will be making. Also, by having you keep the same record this week, you will both be able to see how your energy requirements differ. It will help you both to have a general idea of what your partner should eat relative to what you eat. If you are one of those fortunates who maintains his actual weight close to an ideal weight, it will be helpful to your partner to see how you do that in terms of your calorie intake and output habits. If you are overweight yourself, the record will be helpful to you in seeing why.

If your partner is shifting from a structured diet to a calorie counting approach, she is calculating a daily calorie goal in order to lose a gradual one to two pounds per week. Sit down together and estimate from your diary a daily calorie goal for your own eating. Use the instructions in this chapter to figure how many calories per day it would take for you to maintain your present weight. Compare your calorie requirements with your partner. Do you require 100, 200, 500, or 1000 more calories to maintain your weight while she is losing? Or maybe you require less.

As long as your partner is monitoring her calorie intake and keeping it at a level that allows a decrease in weight, she can eat any particular food she wants. So, if you see her eating a high-calorie food, she is not necessarily "breaking the diet." If she is in fact mis-eating, it is not helpful for you to criticize her—you can be sure she will feel badly enough about it on her own. Instead, your *encouragement* at the time she is practicing new habits (such as measuring food quantities, recording in her dairy, doing slow eating, putting down utensils between bites, or any other behaviors taught in this book) will provide her with immediate incentives to continue, while the ultimate reward of weight loss will not come until later.

Your support for your partner's effort is an important aid, but her own independent efforts are absolutely essential for ultimate success in long-term weight maintenance. This program stresses independence and self-control, yet it may seem that we are asking her to be dependent on you for praise and help. There is, no doubt, a delicate balance that must be found between independence and cooperation between the two of you. We believe it is cooperation, and not dependence, that is helpful in this effort.

chapter four
WILLPOWER

Let's first review what we have covered up to this point:

1. You have examined your motivation with a written Reasons to Lose list and have begun reading it daily.
2. You have settled into a routine of diary keeping, particularly keeping track of all food intake.
3. You have decided on a diet and determined how you will gradually shift to calorie counting, or you have started in with a calorie control system.
4. You have begun learning calorie values and judging quantities. By learning ten to fifteen new values per week, in about eight to nine weeks you will have learned a brief but relatively complete list of about one hundred foods.

We define self-control as the commitment to change, the awareness of choices, and the possession of skills to carry out chosen actions. The more you are aware of the many possible choices concerning eating and the more skills you have for carrying out choices, the better is your level of self-control. So, self-control is not a single thing like a power of will, but is a combination of abilities *which can be improved.* In one way this concept of control gives you more freedom and, we hope, relief from tension—simply because there are always new choices, new options. You should always take the attitude, "Well, I made a mistake; what went wrong, how can I choose more successfully next time?" In another way, though, this concept of control places the responsibility squarely on *your* shoulders. You must accept not only the freedom to choose but the responsibility to choose. We hope this book will give you a lot in the way of new attitudes and skills, but it should take away some things, too: the myth of a cure, a magical pill, or a diet that will make you slim forever—all almost certainly unreasonable hopes. You will have to work to retrain your attitudes and habits. Unfortunately, for most of us this retraining is a difficult and lengthy task, since we've spent a lifetime learning the habits that now lead to mis-eating. You will need patience and persistence. *But the payoff is tremendous: freedom to enjoy any food and to be free of planned diets.*

Since self-control involves choices and skills in many situations, your new learning cannot follow any simple sequence. We all vary as to our problem areas. Some chapters will strike close to home for you, and some will be less relevant.

One way to group our problems is to think of the choice to *start* eating and the choice to *stop*. In the *start* category, we will talk about such issues as tuning in to *real* hunger, knowing how emotions lead you to start eaing, planning your activities and your eating to deal with high temptation or problem times, being assertive with people who urge you to eat, and so forth.

The remainder of this chapter will expand your *start* controls in several ways.

STRATEGIES FOR "START CONTROL"

Your diaries have given you a lot of valuable information about hunger and mis-eating—that is, times when you start eating without being really hungry. We will now discuss strategies to deal with the urge to start mis-eating.

Tolerating Hunger and Delaying Eating

We tend to view hunger as pain, a danger signal to warn us that the body must have food or die. The longer we go without eating, the worse the pain. *Not true.* To the extent that we are animals, hunger does serve this signal purpose. But remember that other animals go out and hunt when they feel hungry, a process that can take hours or days. As civilized humans, food is almost always readily available in our affluent society. The need for our hunger signals has decreased and, therefore, their effectiveness has decreased. Most of us seldom feel really hungry; as a result, we misunderstand or even fear the signals our bodies give us.

It would be useful for you to investigate your own feelings and patterns of hunger. These physical sensations which are your individual hunger pattern are not necessarily painful; more important, they do not get uniformly stronger and stronger with time. If you have ever fasted, whether for a day or longer, you probably noticed that hunger waxes and wanes, like sleepiness. If you are used to eating breakfast, you probably notice hunger soon after arising. If you then skip breakfast, that hunger often goes away and doesn't return for several hours. People who normally skip breakfast are just as empty in the morning as those who eat a big breakfast. They either do not perceive that emptiness as hunger or they intentionally ignore it.

We are *not* recommending that you begin skipping breakfast, but we would like you to experiment with your own hunger sensations to see exactly how they feel, when they occur, and how they change with time. Choose a day when you feel physically well, or reasonably so, and have no special stresses that you know about, and *try* not eating. If you are going to be working or driving a car, a small glass of juice in the morning and every three or four hours will keep you from feeling light-headed. Drink as much of any other low-calorie liquid as you want to, but notice what liquids (especially warm ones) do to your hunger. Note on your diary when the hunger gets stronger, and what happens when you override the hunger and resist eating. Note how different situations affect hunger. You may or may not want to use brief fasts as a tool to control weight at some time in the future. *The point of this exercise is simply to learn about hunger.* We hope that you will notice several things:

1. Hunger is not a terrible pain, but simply a sensation in your

body. You can respond to it by eating or you can ignore it. If you ignore it, it often goes away for a while.

2. What's even more interesting is that the sensation of hunger can be enjoyable. In addition to the pride you feel about being able to resist eating, you may find that hunger gives you a light, energetic feeling. Try it, you may like it!

3. By only drinking juices and not eating for a day, you'll notice much more clearly the rhythm of your body—when hunger comes and goes. This will help you plan a more effective eating schedule.

4. What outside things (sights, smells) cause your hunger to seem to increase?

5. Even if hunger is uncomfortable, by not eating you'll learn what kinds of other activities are effective distractions. For example, you may find that mental activity is difficult when you're hungry, but a brisk walk completely takes your mind off it. If you feel very uncomfortable and light-headed, drink some juice.

Record your self-observations for the day you choose to go without eating on the Diary Notes side of your weekly diary.

On the other days, each time you get the urge to snack, delay for ten minutes and then decide whether and what to eat. If you choose not to eat the snack, note that on your diary too (with a star next to the note). Again, note what kinds of activities help you to delay. Is there a mental phrase that helps? For example, try saying to yourself, "It's mine, and I can have it later."

Some of you will try fasting for a day and not notice any signs of hunger. We don't want you to continue fasting beyond one day. Frequently, people who don't feel hunger are those whose eating is irregular and who often go for fairly long periods without eating. It is important to sense hunger after several hours of fasting. If you are one of those people who do not feel hunger, one way to regain that sensitivity is to spend a period of time eating very regularly, three meals a day at the usual times. After a week to two weeks of this, try the one-day fast again. You will probably then be much more aware of hunger sensations. After that you can decide again whether you want to continue on a regular meal pattern or return to a more irregular pattern, perhaps then based on eating when you really feel hungry.

CONTROLLING YOURSELF BY CONTROLLING YOUR OWN ENVIRONMENT

Most of us believe self-control to be a kind of mental "grit your teeth." Food or the thought of food seems to pull at us until we eventually give in. We prefer to define self-control, in more practical terms, as all of the skills we use to make choices when we experience a conflict, in this case about eating. It is important to recognize that although it feels as if we are resisting or not resisting eating by our inner will, we are often being very much affected by the immediate environment around us. Experiments have shown that many overweight people are especially sensitive to their environment, eating more in response to outside events than in response to internal sensations of hunger. For example, in one study, obese and nonobese people were given a task to do over a period of several hours. The experimenter secretly moved the clock in the room gradually forward more quickly than normal, so that "lunchtime" occurred earlier. Those who were obese were more likely to eat when the clock said it was lunchtime, and they ate more than the nonobese people, proving their greater vulnerability to the clock.

Although control of eating may be partly in the environment, self-control—as we have defined it—can include changing your own environment. You don't have to be a passive victim of the environment, but can take self-control by reshaping your environment so that you are less tempted to mis-eat.

Shopping and Preparation

Self-control is always time-related. The more steps you can take in advance of the time when you are confronted with the choice to eat, the easier it will be to avoid mis-eating. Grocery shopping is one of the earliest steps that you can modify to make later choices easier. Here are a few suggestions:

1. Try to shop from a list rather than by walking up and down the aisles, letting the packages attract you. Become aware of how

packages do affect you; they're intentionally designed to appeal to your eyes. Look for packages that have a number of individual packages inside, so that you will have less food exposed at home, making it harder to casually use up what's available in a large container. Be aware of the growing number of packages that contain calorie information on the label. Start to shop wisely in terms of calorie cost, just as you do in terms of dollar cost. For example, plain yogurt is about 160 calories for a one-cup container. If you add your own fresh fruit or even a teaspoon of jam, your calorie total is lower than the 250–320 calories for flavored yogurts.

2. Notice which times of day for shopping are better for your self-control. Some people find that they buy less when they're very hungry (because they're in a hurry to get home to eat). Others buy more when they're hungry (everything looks tempting). See which category fits you, and try to plan your shopping accordingly.

3. In writing your shopping list, try to plan in terms of actual menus. You should aim toward well-planned, attractively prepared meals, rather than being forced into using fast convenience foods which may be higher in calories. If you are very busy or often don't enjoy cooking, perhaps you can use your freezer compartment to have available some well-balanced, lower-calorie meals. There are many good, low-calorie cookbooks on the market. Experiment with new dishes. The basic rule is to enjoy your food, but if you can find lower-calorie good foods you like, then you're that much ahead.

Organizing Your Kitchen and Pantry

If you have high-calorie foods around, either because you choose to eat them in moderation or because other members of the household do, keep them in a separate cupboard or on a separate shelf. While you don't need to play the game of locking up or hiding foods, isolating them will allow you to make clear and conscious choices about these foods. Any step that makes temptation easier to resist, will build your self-control.

Signs and Posters

Visual reminders are very helpful. For example, your isolated, high-calorie foods can bear a sign saying "Beware." Past clients of ours have made up stop signs, much like the eight-sided traffic signs, and placed them on the refrigerator. Signs can also be used to remind yourself to do some of the new self-control techniques you're learning (for example, "Don't forget your diary"). These reminders tend to blend into the surroundings and lose their effectiveness over time, so it's important to change them around to attract your attention.

Restrict Where You Eat

From now on, make it a rule that you will do *all* of your at-home eating sitting down in either your kitchen or dining room. Even if it's a small snack, go to a regular eating place for it. No more eating in front of the TV, or in bed, or standing in front of the refrigerator!

Generally, try not to be distracted while you are eating. Eating with other people and having conversation are fine, but *don't watch TV or read*. When you eat, really eat! Concentrate and enjoy.

Those of you who eat alone may find this difficult. Try it for a few days, and see if you don't eat less and get used to restricting your activity this way. The converse of this rule is useful too: Don't do other activities around food. If you use the kitchen table to study or do some other work, you're more likely to snack while you do the other activity. If at all possible, stay out of the kitchen except when preparing food, eating, or cleaning up. If a family member asks for a snack, urge him to prepare his own and eat it out of your sight unless you plan to join him. In Chapter 14 we discuss in detail the family and other social pressures related to eating.

Packaging Your Own Snacks

Foods often are not packaged in sizes designed to help your self-control. As we indicated earlier, food manufacturers are oriented toward increasing, not decreasing, consumption. It will be worth your effort to preplan snacks by wrapping foods in small, snack-size packages—each labeled as to number of calories. If you know you will want a snack at a regular time, you can label a snack package with the date and time for consumption. The effort involved in unwrapping small packages of food may be enough to limit your snack on many occasions. This is especially true for foods that are not ordinarily packaged (like one slice of bread or two crackers). Knowing that you have ready an acceptable "Tuesday, 11 P.M. snack" can decrease the conflict over eating at other times in the evening.

Setting the Table and Sitting Down to Eat

It's important that your food and your table setting be as attractive as possible. If you are preparing lower-calorie foods, prepare them in as attractive and tasty a form as you can. You might consider buying yourself your own special place mat which you put under your table setting each time you eat, even if it's only a snack. Again, being formal and being aware increases self-control.

Try to avoid putting serving plates full of food on your table. Serve yourself the portion you have decided to eat, and leave the rest in containers away from the table. There are two considerations about keeping food warm. On the one hand, you might find that taking the total portion you want to allow yourself and then letting any leftovers get cold may discourage taking seconds. The alternative strategy is to deliberately take a smaller portion, but to keep the rest warm so that you know you can have more later. This takes the pressure off and allows you to make another choice when later comes along and you may be feeling less hungry. Try both approaches, and see which works best. You may find one better with certain foods, but not others.

When you sit down to eat, count and record the calories you've served yourself *before you start eating*, if possible. This will help to insure that you are taking responsibility and making choices.

Finally, try this trick on your eyes: Serve your meal on a smaller plate. Spread the food to cover the plate, and use the smallest plate that seems reasonable (for example, a salad or luncheon plate instead of a dinner plate). We tend to fill our plates and to feel cheated when the food looks lost on a large plate, so the smaller plate does have a pronounced psychological advantage.

After Meals

The conflict over whether to start eating again after a meal is over is a common one for many people. Although you may later want to practice tolerating presence of food at the end of a meal, it's probably best at this stage to leave the table as soon as you've finished your meal—or better yet, as soon as you begin to feel satisfied and can leave some food. If you're responsible for cleaning up, try to have company around if you're one of those people who nibbles on the scraps. It's interesting how each of us defines garbage. For some, food on our own plates left for a few minutes loses its appeal and won't be touched. Others have no problem eating cold scraps on our own plates, but wouldn't think of eating from someone else's plate. Still others would eat from a family member's or close friend's plate, but not from a stranger's plate. For some, the definition centers on location—nibbling leftovers is okay at the table, but never at the sink. Finally, there are a few who are able to eat leftovers that have been discarded in a trash or garbage can. What's your definition of garbage?

Many of us like to linger at the table and enjoy conversation, perhaps over coffee. Try having the coffee at some other location, or completely clearing the table except for coffee.

The rule that should be observed as strictly as possible is, "This place is for enjoying eating; don't associate it with other activities that may lead to mis-eating."

SPECIAL "START" PROBLEMS

You have already begun your path to better start control by keeping diaries. Eventually, counting calories will give you a record of your intake that will be invaluable for start control. The key word is *information*. You cannot make a choice without information. By knowing what your calorie total should average and how much you've taken in at any given time of day, you have information essential in the choice of whether to start eating and, if so, what kind and amount of food you can plan. Your food diary can be your budget, checkbook, and bank statement all rolled into one. It will help you not only to plan a given day and to choose whether to *start* at any particular time, but will allow you to take the past and future into account. For example, if you want to average 1200 calories daily and you know you're going to a dinner party on Friday, you can save up calories for several days to prepare for a splurge—100 calories less on Tuesday, Wednesday, and Thursday should allow for a special dessert on Friday. Like some recent bank checking accounts, your food diary also allows you to "go into the red"; that is, if you overeat by a given amount on one day, you know how much you should pay back on the following few days to get even and achieve your calorie average for the week. While saving is better than borrowing, the system allows for both. Again, freedom means responsibility. You can no longer say, "I blew my diet, so I might as well forget the whole thing" and then continue overeating. You need not fast nor even radically cut back on the following days. Instead, you can *gradually* pay back the calories you overate.

Take a sheet of paper and divide it with a line down the middle. Head the left-hand column "Problem Times" and the right-hand column "Solutions." You're going to list the problem times you can think of and work out as many alternative solutions as possible. First list any problems related to time—either time of day, time of week, or time of month. If you have to have problems, these are the best kind, because they recur with predictable regularity. "Every afternoon I eat while I make dinner." "Every evening I munch while I watch television." "Saturday nights I eat candy at the movies." "Sunday brunch I eat sweet rolls." "Just before my period I go crazy for chocolates."

We'll now give you some planned strategies for these examples, but you are in the best position to devise your own actual solutions. Our persistent message is for you to focus on self-help and independence; your own solutions will work best for you. Have at least two alternate strategies, experimenting until you find the best one; post the sheet where you can see it to remind you of what needs to be done.

One type of solution to the time-related problem is based on what you have learned in this chapter about delaying—that is, finding a strategy to help you tolerate the hunger and get past the hunger period.

Let's look at the late-afternoon nibbler. She may come home from work at five, tired and tense, be faced with children and their problems, and expect to get a dinner ready for her husband's arrival at 6:00. A possible solution involves assertiveness and relaxation. She can tell her family that her *real* arrival time is 5:30, and that from 5:00 to 5:30 she is unavailable except for emergencies (real ones!). During this time she relaxes in whatever way suits her individual preference—lying down, napping, having a bubble bath, reading, puttering in the garden, meditating, or simply doing nothing. She may also find it necessary to assert herself in getting the family's help in preparing dinner. The relaxation will reduce hunger and also give her more energy to be with the family for the rest of the evening.

A completely different solution could involve calorie budgeting. This woman could try allotting two hundred calories for an "arrival snack," something enjoyable to tide her over to dinner (for example, a small glass of wine and an ounce of cheese).

A similar time-related solution can be used for the premenstrual chocolate fancier. That is, if she can predict those days by marking the calendar, she can reserve some calories in her budget, prepackage and label some chocolate, eat the chocolate slowly, with great enjoyment, and not have to feel one bit of guilt. Premenstrual tension can also be relieved in other ways by planning some relaxing and pleasurable events for those days. If the tension is severe, you may want to consult a physician.

Another timing solution involves eating to prevent miseating. This is a good one to help the "candy at the movies" problem. A simple strategy is to be sure to eat a light meal within your calorie budget just before the movies. You can also take along your own movie snack to foil owner's offering of giant-sized candy bars. Your snack could be a lower-calorie alternative to chocolate, or it could be a premeasured, safe amount of chocolate.

Here are some examples of problem times and their possible solutions. They were given to us by our clients and are presented here in their own words.

Problem	Solutions
1. Very tense every afternoon 3:30–5:30 due to hungry kids and my short temper. Nibble while cooking.	a. Prepare nutritious snack for kids to get after naps and have a juice break for myself around 4 P.M.
	b. Go for a walk if I don't have much dinner preparation to do.
	c. Practice the slow, deep breathing that relaxed me during childbirths.
	d. Have vegetable juice beforehand. Allow the children to assist in the preparations. Play music as a reminder of the outside world.
	e. Chew gum while in the kitchen.
	f. Have a cup of tea to sip while I cook.
2. Weekends are sometimes difficult when our extended family gets together and an impromptu meal is suggested, such as going out for pizza or hamburgers.	a. Try to budget enough calories to enjoy.
	b. Limit portion sizes.
	c. Eat slowly.
	d. Talk more.
3. Eating in the evening.	a. Budget calories and prepare snack packages.
	b. Organize a corner for activities away from kitchen.
	c. Post favorite-activity list there.
	d. Get out of house (e.g., walk).
4. Every Sunday I get up early, before my husband, have breakfast and read the paper, then have breakfast again with him.	a. Get up when husband gets up.
	b. If I get up early, have a plan of something to do: Write letters, wash, etc., and delay breakfast until he is up.
	c. Get up early, have juice and coffee with paper. Save toast and eggs to have with him.

Problem	*Solutions*
5. Every weekend when I do my big grocery shopping, I stop off somewhere for a snack or eat some cookies while I am shopping.	a. Plan shopping *directly after lunch*. b. Plan something nice to do at home so I will whiz through the shopping and get home as fast as I can.
6. Every day I am tempted to eat goodies at morning coffee break.	a. Go for a walk instead of going with others at break. b. Keep working at my desk and don't join others. c. *Be sociable*, but stick to coffee. (Put sign in my change purse to remind me: "Nothing but coffee," then think of all the calories saved).
7. On weekends, while out shopping, I can't resist eating out, especially junk food, (ice cream, hot dogs, hamburgers, candy, Cokes.)	a. Allow myself to buy one favorite food, eat only half and throw rest away. Include in daily calorie count.
8. Celebrations—birthday parties for the family, holiday meals, etc.	a. Under-eat during the week before and after. b. Reduce size of helpings of birthday cake, etc. c. Hold each bite in my mouth longer so that my small portions take as long to eat as the others' large portions.
9. Desire for dessert or something sweet to end a meal.	a. Eat fruit. b. End the meal with a Tic Tac breath mint. Mint satisfies my sweet tooth fairly well.
10. Rushing at too fast a pace in office, then eating out of frustration, fast and furiously snacking.	a. Use cot room for a five-minute rest. b. Take a ten-minute relaxation break to slow down.

SUGGESTED PARTNER ACTIVITY

The major task for your partner in shopping, organizing the food cupboards, and eating out is to make decisions in advance about what foods to choose, and then to arrange the environment to help discourage yielding to temptation. Your partner may decide to make significant changes in her way of grocery shopping, her food storage, and her snacking habits. You can help her by becoming aware of these reorganizing efforts which she feels will help her gain control over the constant pulls toward eating in her daily life. You might have some observations about possible changes that would be valuable.

There are numerous possibilities in the topics covered in this chapter, and the two of you will know best about what specific strategies fit your particular life-style. Listed below are some suggestions you might find valuable.

1. Think and talk about where eating (snacking especially) occurs in your house. If you snack while watching TV or reading in bed late at night, is this a temptation time for your partner? If so, you might choose to snack in this way only when your partner is not present to be tempted. A different way to handle this might be for your partner to save extra calories for these snacks and actually prepare exact amounts ahead of time. The two of you need to decide which approach will work for you.

2. If you shop, what should you do about bringing home foods that are just too tempting for your partner right now? Maybe there are particular foods that you will both agree should not be brought home, at least for the present. Perhaps you can use a separate storage area for foods you wish to have at home and which your partner wishes to avoid.

3. Decide on how the pantry should be organized and help your partner put groceries away in their newly designated places.

4. Help by clearing serving dishes with leftover food from the table immediately after finishing the meal. If you help with the cleanup, scrape the leftovers on the plates directly into the garbage in order to help her avoid nibbling.

5. When you go out to eat, plan ahead of time to choose a restaurant with menu selections that will make it easy to keep the calories down. If your partner has trouble being assertive about making requests of the waiter, encourage her to give it a try anyway. If you are good at it, tell her how you do it.

This week your partner is also working on identifying the problem times and circumstances that lead to mis-eating for her. Think about whether or not any such circumstances ever lead you to mis-eat. Many people who don't have problems with overweight mis-eat too when they feel sad, tired, or angry, or when they are around others who are eating a lot. The fact that these people do not develop weight problems, while others do, can be the consequence of several factors. People with a genetic tendency toward overweight will need to control their mis-eating if they want to control their weight. Other people who mis-eat may do it so infrequently that no weight gain occurs. If you ever mis-eat, you have an eating problem similar at times to your partner's.

If you do not have a mis-eating problem, you might handle tension in a different way that is also not profitable. For instance, you may smoke when you're tense or withdraw from contact with others when you are feeling low. If you have more constructive ways of dealing with problems that your wife copes with by mis-eating, it might help her if you would share these with her. Keep in mind that what will work for her might be quite different than what works for you.

Sometime this week, talk with your partner about her analysis of situations that lead her to mis-eat. Maybe you have noticed mis-eating times for her that she hasn't. Maybe you have solution strategies that would be helpful and maybe you could be directly involved in helping her through some of the difficult times. For instance, if evening eating is a problem, you could accompany your partner on a walk as she attempts to get away from the refrigerator.

Again, it is important to remember that there is a balance between independence and dependence in your partner's attempt to learn self-control. You can help her come to solutions for mis-eating; you can help by eating slowly, being a good model and good company at meals; you can help by praising or reinforcing her practice of new eating behaviors and by being noncritical in your response to her mis-eating. But you cannot take over and do what is necessary for her to do. If you try, you might have a rebellion on your hands.

chapter five
STOP CONTROL

Self-control is a matter of choices: choosing when and where to eat, choosing what and how to eat, and choosing when to stop. One of the problems in relying on structured diets is that they don't help you learn when to stop.

Some people have a natural, built-in, hunger-and-satisfaction control system. Their bodies say, "You're hungry—eat" or "You've had enough—stop." Most overweight and formerly overweight people lack that automatic physical control system. It can be improved by practicing certain techniques we will teach you, and it can be supplemented by mental controls. If your body doesn't tell you when to stop, your head can remind you. For example, you will feel more full twenty minutes to a half hour after finishing a meal. Therefore, if you eat until you're just satisfied, you will feel comfortably full in a half hour. If, on the other hand, you eat until you are full, you will feel stuffed in a half hour. You may remember that uncomfortable feeling after you have gotten into the car, following a dinner out in a restaurant. How often have you said, "I wish I hadn't had that second helping" or "If only I had passed up dessert"? If you stop *before* you are full, you will feel just right in a very short time. You should be eating until you are satisfied instead of eating until you are full. As you practice stopping, the distinction between these two feelings will become clearer.

One important technique in retuning your body to recognize hunger and satisfaction and in giving your mind a chance to control your hands and mouth is to *slow down* the whole process. Our research has shown that overweight people tend to eat faster than thin people. So, your first lesson in *how* to eat is to slow down. Here are the steps for a demonstration that will help you to experience the benefits of slower eating.

1. Make sure you haven't eaten for at least three or four hours, but are not so ravenous that you are unable to relax and try the exercise. Make sure you'll have at least a half hour of privacy without distraction.

2. Get *half* an apple (or similar fruit, if your prefer), a glass with four ounces of liquid (such as fruit juice), and a straw.

3. Sit down and close your eyes. Notice any physical signs of hunger and/or thirst. These may be the traditional rumbling of the tummy or may involve some other sensations, such as a generally empty feeling, tension in the neck, dryness of the throat, slight headache, or even slight nausea or light-headedness.

4. Pick up the apple, look at it carefully, sniff it, and then take a *small* bite—but leave it *unchewed* in your mouth.

5. Move the piece of apple around in your mouth. Notice the texture against your tongue and cheek.

6. Begin to chew very slowly. Allow a full thirty seconds to chew this bite slowly, swallowing as little as possible until the end. Notice all the aspects of the chewing: the texture of the skin and meat of the apple, the taste of the juice, the coolness of it against your teeth, the feeling as it goes down your throat into your stomach. Try to experience this eating as fully as possible; close your eyes while chewing.

7. Rest for fifteen seconds before taking another small bite and repeating the slow chewing. Remember to put the apple down between bites.

8. After about four bites, and when your mouth is cleared of food, slowly take a sip of liquid. Now stop and close your eyes and reexamine your hunger sensations. Notice any changes. Do you feel less hungry?

9. Take more bites, slowly, followed by sips of liquid between bites, only if you still notice any signs of hunger. Check in with yourself frequently and ask yourself whether you are still hungry. Stop as soon as you feel no more hunger signs. Now throw away the rest of the apple and juice.

10. Repeat this exercise once a day for a week. Generally, try to slow down your eating at meals. Here are a few tips on doing this.

> Pause before you start a meal. Consciously say to yourself, "Slow down and enjoy." Do whatever you can to make each meal a relaxed experience—listen to pleasant music, avoid tense discussions.
>
> Stop for thirty seconds mid-meal and repeat the phrase, "Slow down and enjoy."
>
> As often as possible, put down your utensils or hand-held food while you are still chewing what's in your mouth. Some people find it helpful to shift the fork periodically to the "wrong" hand; the awkwardness slows you down. *Focus on the flavor of the food.*
>
> Avoid distractions like TV or reading while you eat.
>
> Drink between bites, not with food in your mouth. A drink, especially something warm before the meal, may reduce hunger considerably.

Using these techniques (and any others you can think of), try to extend as many meals as you can by at least ten minutes. There are many skills you can learn to develop what we will call "stop control." The first important step to achieving stop control is learning to eat slowly and sensuously. Slowing down will enable you to be more aware of sensations of hunger and satisfaction. Eating slowly puts you in touch with your body. It puts you in the driver's seat and gives you control of the brakes as well as the accelerator.

Notice that what we are referring to as slow eating can take different forms—e.g., actually chewing each mouthful slowly or chewing at your usual rate but stopping periodically. The goal is to increase your awareness of the process of eating, to enjoy it more, but also to insist that your conscious self recognizes what you're consuming and makes choices. Whether we are simply distracted or are unconsciously identifying with a nurturing mother by feeding ourselves instead of actively eating, the result is a loss of a sense of control and a higher likelihood of mis-eating.

STOP CLEANING YOUR PLATE

This is an area of utmost importance when so often we are faced with more food than we can afford to eat (especially when someone else serves us.). While we have begun to show you how slower, more aware eating will help you notice satisfaction sooner, we must face the reality that often the choice to stop is not based on the absence of hunger. You can go on eating for any of a number of reasons: because of a sense of social obligation, the pleasure of taste in your mouth, the nonhunger tensions in your body, or just from sheer habit. It will take a conscious effort to change your attitude about leaving food and learning some skills to enable you to choose to stop.

Great quantities of food are wasted in our society. People are starving in other parts of the world. Probably your mother taught you to "clean your plate"; and probably you do just that most of the time.

It's time to stop cleaning your plate. It's not helping the starving of the world. It's not even helping your pocketbook, since it contributes to your overeating. The best way to break this habit is with a kind of self-shock treatment for a few days. We want you to experience throwing away some perfectly good food. Prepare a normal-size plateful of food for yourself at mealtime. Sit down with the plate in front of you. Divide each food in half with your fork. Get up, go to the sink or garbage can, and throw half away! Watch it go down the drain or close the lid to the can, and sit down again. Notice all of your feelings about doing this. Make some notes in your diary. Go on and eat the rest of your meal. Eat slowly, savor and enjoy the food. This exercise is designed to give you the first experience of not eating all of the food you serve yourself or which is served to you. The small amount of food wasted will be worthwhile in the long run because this will help you to learn to eat less. The exercise is not designed to deprive you of food for that day. If, *after at least an hour*, you're still hungry, go back and eat something else.

Do this exercise once a day for three days. If our past experience is correct, many of you will find this a painful, if not impossible, task to perform. Your conscience screams, "Waste not; people are starving. This is a sin." We can only insist again that *if you haven't tried it, you should*, for two reasons: It will force you to examine all of the irrational ideas and fears you have about wasting food, and it will prepare you for the next step in controlling stopping. No one will starve, least of all you; you won't be struck by lightning. We hope you will lose a bit of your reverence for food; you'll realize that you do have enough.

Then, on to Step 2. Again, for one meal a day, we want you to divide each food on the plate in half, so that you can see a clear dividing line. Begin eating. When you reach the dividing line, stop and consciously make the decision *not* to go on. As quickly as possible, then, get the food out of your sight. This time you can put the leftovers away for another time if you want to. Leave the table. If you're hungry *(at least an hour later)*, you may eat something else. This is an exercise in stopping; *it's not designed to cut your calories for the day*. Do not take an extra-large or a double portion for this exercise. Be fair. No one will cheat you out of what's due. Be aware of any feelings of being cheated or deprived in this situation. But also be aware of any feelings of pride at being able to stop. Stopping is perhaps even more important, and more difficult, than start control. There are so many times when we take or are given more food on our plates than we honestly want to eat. Hunger changes as you start into a meal. Yet you feel compelled to eat it all, either out of conscience, habit, or courtesy. In the long run your waistline, your pocketbook, the economy, and the world's starving masses will all benefit from the ability to stop and really not waste.

After you've had three days of throwing half a plate of food away before a meal (once a day), followed by three days of pre-dividing the food and stopping at the dividing line (storing it for another meal if you wish), you can go one step further in self-control. Try making the choice to stop without predividing the food. When it looks as if you're about halfway through the meal, stop for one minute (time yourself; it helps to actually leave the table) and then ask yourself if you're *really* still hungry. If the answer is no, stop and store the food immediately. If you decide to go on eating, stop before you clean the plate. Leave *at least one forkful* of each food on the plate—again, get rid of the food as soon as you decide to stop. Practice this stopping exercise at least once a day.

Continue to try to leave one or several forkfuls of food at each meal. You will be pleasantly surprised at the bonus you will have in calories saved. As you do this stopping exercise, each time you leave a forkful of food, try to figure out how many calories you chose not to eat.

Notice on the calorie chart that we have provided an extra column for small amounts of each food. For example, potato chips are two hundred calories for a small bag. We figured *each potato chip* is about ten calories. That information might help you leave one potato chip in the bag and save ten calories. (It might even help you to decide to eat only one potato chip!)

As you begin leaving a small amount of food, like one spoonful or one forkful, begin to fill in the calorie amount for the small amounts in that extra column. It will come in handy to know how many calories are in one bite of hamburger sandwich!

We noted in Chapter 4 that getting away from the table after a meal is important to avoid starting to eat again. In this chapter we have focused on the process of stopping before your plate is clean. In social eating, especially if there are serving dishes on the table, the definition of the end of eating is sometimes unclear. Coffee, cigarettes, after-dinner alcoholic drinks all serve to define the end of eating. The definition is social, psychological, and physiological. Once these activities begin, going back to the food available on your plate or on the table is more difficult; it is a bit embarrassing and the food tends to taste less desirable. You can look for your own effective pattern of meal enders. French gourmets and wine experts speak of "clearing the palate." A sweet, a liqueur, a cigarette, even a drink of water, or a sharp-tasting fruit like a slice of lemon can change your taste sensations enough to help you to stop. One client of ours told us that she regularly brushed her teeth when she was having trouble stopping.

Here's a final point about stopping. You may remember that we said one of the purposes of the exercise in throwing away food was to reduce your reverence for food so that you'll feel less compelled to eat everything put in front of you. Here are some things you might want to try to help you let go of those special feelings for food:

1. Cook or bake or buy some food to give away to someone else. Give it without eating any yourself. Make it clear that it's a gift and that you'd rather not eat any (the person receiving the gift should not be overweight!)

2. Play with some food. Take some bread and wad it up with a little water until it's a spongy glob. You can mold it into different shapes. Or just run your fingers through some food that you're going to throw away anyway, just to see how it feels.

3. Play a creativity game, perhaps with others in your family. It goes like this: List all of the crazy uses you can think of for a cookie or some other food (wheels for a midget car, paperweights for tissue paper, hockey pucks for soft hockey sticks).

DEVELOPING AWARE EATING FURTHER

We would like you to focus in detail on your experience of eating. Don't make any special effort to change or to do it all correctly right now. Just notice what happens, and make some notes in your diary about such things as:

1. How does your hunger change from before a meal to during and after a meal?
2. Are there any feelings of tension before, during, or after (where do you notice them in your body)?
3. Are there differences between meals in your sense of control over eating (time of day, who is with you)?
4. How do you try to slow down your eating? Which techniques work best?
5. What distractions are hardest to avoid (reading, TV)? How do you go on automatic pilot (your hand feeding your mouth almost as if it belongs to someone else)?
6. For which foods or which meals are you able to leave some food on your plate? How does it feel to do this?

RATE YOUR AWARENESS AND CONTROL

Our goal is to help you to personalize *aware eating*, to develop a style that works for you. Some of the techniques will be better than others for you. The important point will be to increase your sense of control of your eating and to increase your ability to get more enjoyment from smaller quantities.

As a step toward this goal, we would like you to rate each meal or snack as to the degree of this sense of control, awareness, and enjoyment. Give a score of 5 to an especially aware and enjoyable meal or snack, 3 to an average meal or snack, and 1 to a meal or snack that seemed to be especially tense, hurried, or unsatisfying. (You can use 4's and 2's on the scale for anything that is in between.) For the next week, place this rating on the Food Diary next to the foods eaten at that time, and circle the number. By comparing your ratings with your diary notes on the questions listed just above, you will begin to see which components lead to that sense of aware, controlled, satisfying eating. Then you will be able to selectively practice those techniques that will work for you and also see if your rating numbers go up more frequently.

TALK TO YOURSELF

To close this chapter, we would like to suggest a principle and a new technique that may be useful to some of you.

It is helpful to organize your thoughts and get them expressed openly. This is why we stress the importance of your diary notes; they serve as a release and source of information for you, as well as a way for you to get to know your problems better. Often we think a lot about ourselves and our problems, with thoughts and associated feelings going round and round in our heads. Actually saying or writing those thoughts can be a relief from preoccupation and a way to get a greater clarity about yourself and what you want to do. Some of you have done this with diary notes and found it beneficial. Others have various ways to accomplish the same goal (talking with a close friend or a counselor, writing in your own diary, etc.)

If you are someone who could benefit from this activity, we urge you to write more. It may be important that you get those thoughts and feelings out.

As a supplement to writing, you may want to consider a new technique: talking to a tape recorder. Many people these days have an inexpensive cassette recorder, but wouldn't think of using it this way. Set aside a regular time each day, find a private place, and *talk to your tape recorder* (you can also cry to it, scream at it, or laugh into it). Say anything that comes into your head. Practice not censoring yourself. Whether or not you ever listen to what you said is of secondary importance; just saying it will help. You can even erase it immediately afterward. This is a concrete way to develop further your sense of independence; you can be your own friend and help yourself. It doesn't preclude talking or writing to someone else, but can be an important addition.

Finally, consider increasing *aware eating* by talking to your food. At the risk of sounding loony if caught, a number of our clients have effectively increased their control over food by saying (aloud when they're alone) such things as: "You're not worth the calories," "I won't give in to you," "I love you, but we can't go on meeting like this."

SUGGESTED PARTNER ACTIVITY

Your partner is beginning to practice ways of slowing down her eating. When you sit down to eat with her at your meals this week, both of you should notice whether you eat faster, slower, or at the same rate. If you tend to eat more slowly than your mate, then she can try to match her eating pace to yours.

Slower eating makes meals more pleasant and satisfying, once you get used to the relaxed pace. In general, anything you do to make mealtimes more pleasant for the two of you will increase eating satisfaction for both of you.

Your partner's lesson this week also includes the first exercise in developing stop controls. She is going to deal with the reactions within herself that will come from actually throwing away half a plate of food. Try this with her at the first meal you have together this week and note your own reactions to the exercise. Do you feel deprived, or do you feel it's a shame to waste good food? Is it a tolerable or intolerable thing to do? The shock tactic of this exercise is very effective in beginning to develop stop controls. The initial discomforts with the exercise must be considered in view of the long-range alteration of eating habits.

chapter six
"I HATE EXERCISE"

From the beginning of this program we have asked you to record your physical activity and exercise in your diary. We feel strongly about increasing energy output at the same time that you decrease food intake.

Let's first review the main facts about the energy balance of your body. You take in potential energy in the form of food. The amount of energy in a given food is measured in calories. A calorie is actually a measure of the amount of heat energy that would be released if you burned the food (for calorie books they figure it out by burning the food in a kind of furnace). Your body works roughly like a furnace or the engine of a car; the food is slowly burned for moving the body around and for producing heat. If your body's energy system is perfectly in balance, you are taking in the same amount as you are burning. If you take in too much, the excess is stored as fat (like an expandable gas tank). If you take in too little, you use up the fuel (fat) in storage. This means that you lose fat by taking in less, or by using up more.

If you stayed in bed all day you would still use up energy (for working internal organs, generating heat, breathing). The amount used in this way varies according to body size and characteristics of your body engine (your gas mileage, so to speak). The average woman burns about 1400 calories per day without even moving.

Every activity burns up more calories. Unfortunately, in our society we tend more and more to move less and less, what with cars, elevators, and other appliances.

It seems clear from this analysis that you can lose weight by increasing your activity. First let's look at some of the myths about physical activity and exercise and some of the advantages.

It takes, on the average, 3500 calories of extra activity to use up a pound of fat (i.e., beyond what you do to burn the food you're eating). If you burn five calories a minute in a moderately fast walk and walk a mile in twenty minutes, that figures out to one hundred calories per mile, or walking thirty-five miles to lose a pound. Not worth it, you say. View these facts another way, however. If you were to add *twenty minutes* of walking daily, you would lose ten pounds a year with no other effort or reduction in food intake. So, even this moderate exercise would be a great help to a weight-reduction program and especially to a weight-maintenance program.

"But exercise works up your appetite," you say. "Why bother, if I'll eat up even more afterward than I burned?" A myth! Many studies indicate that the *opposite* is true. *In*activity leads to increased appetite. Just think about how ranchers raise cattle. When they want to fatten them up, they put them in pens away from the open range. There they overeat. Similar observations show that at summer camps, the overweight children exercise less and eat more. Professional athletes will also attest to the fact that they feel *less* hungry after a strenuous physical workout. Most telling, though, is your own experience. Most of you recognize that when you are less active, when you stay at home, you get bored and eat more.

Another myth to explode is that exercise is painful or unpleasant. We like to use the words *physical activity*. One of our clients wrote that she hated exercise, but loved to play tennis. A retired man wrote to say he strongly disliked exercise, but first on his list of pleasures was his daily two-hour walk! Increasing your physical activity does not have to mean doing *unpleasant* exercises. Calisthenics are fine only if you really *enjoy* doing them. Is window shopping unpleasant? Is playing with your kids painful? Is sex unpleasant? *All activity* is exercise in the sense that it burns calories.

You only need to find the level and type of activity that suits you.

Finally, here are some facts about exercise that correct some other common myths:

> Passive exercise (by machines) and massage may be pleasant, but they don't take off weight.
>
> Sweating (by sauna or steam) produces only a temporary loss due to loss of fluid.
>
> Spot reducing is generally not possible. You can tighten stomach muscles, but you can generally expect to lose fat all over and maintain your same proportions when you lose weight, by whatever means. If you have big hips and thighs, they will get smaller, but will still be relatively big compared to the rest of you.
>
> Of course, sex burns calories. You might make it a part of your family conference (Chapter 14) to discuss ways to increase this form of calorie output.

Just to finish our argument in favor in physical activity, here is a list of the advantages:

1. Activity burns calories. In addition to the statistics described above, you should be aware of what we call our "tip the balance" theory. We have found that when your energy intake and output is almost in balance (you're neither gaining nor losing) a slight shift in favor of a deficit in calories (for example, by burning only one hundred calories more per day through activity) tips the balance, and you'll lose a pound or two per week. This is not proven, but seems to happen frequently.

2. Physical activity is a great substitute and distracter at times of temptation to mis-eat. Also, as we've said, vigorous activity actually reduces appetite for a while.

3. Physical activity is an antidepressant. It really does help to chase away the blues.

4. Physical activity tones the muscles, speeds up size loss (especially in the waist) as weight loss progresses, and helps you feel better about your body image.

5. Physical activity generally improves your sense of well-being, your feeling of energy, and your health.

So much for the sales pitch. Now, how do you go about it? The first key word is *gradually*. Know your limits; check with a physician if you have any doubts; then, gradually increase your output. Begin with fifty calories of additional activity a day. As soon as you feel comfortable, increase it by another fifty. Try a goal this week of boosting your output by fifty to one hundred calories a day. Record all new activity on your Physical Activity Diary. The printed form gives you an estimate of calories per minutes for different types of activity.

There are a number of ways to increase your energy output. Simplest—but probably least interesting—is calisthenics or other indoor muscle-toning exercise. There are many good books and classes on this. The Canadian Air Force exercise program is published in a book, is widely acclaimed, and gives you a program of gradually increasing output.

Another important way to increase output is by walking— pleasant, invigorating, and safe because your body will naturally protect you from overdoing it. Also, it's important to look for ways to increase your walking in the context of daily activities: Park your car a block or two away from your destination, get off the elevator a floor away from your destination, walk to the mailbox instead of driving, etc. As you get used to this approach, you'll be putting out more calories each day without even noticing it.

"I hate sports!" "Sports are not for fat people!" Usually the people who say they hate sports are the people who don't participate. It's hard to get started, especially if you're self-conscious about your appearance. But, like so many other habits, once you get over the initial effort, you get hooked. Give yourself a chance. Try different sports until one feels like it might become pleasant. It helps to participate with a friend. Once you are hooked you not only won't hate it, you will feel miserable if you don't get in your round of golf, set of tennis, swimming, or whatever. To get yourself hooked, it may help to reward yourself for participation during the beginning stages (this goes for walking or any other activity). Plan something pleasant (not food!) after the activity.

A few general tips: Do heavier activities on a relatively empty stomach, if possible. Allow yourself at least a half hour after a physical activity before eating. If you've sweated, a liquid (non-calorie), not a food, is what you need. Relax your body between exercise and eating. As much relaxation of muscles as possible before eating will reduce your appetite. Do light physical activity after a meal. A walk in the evening after dinner is not only delightful, it tends to speed up your metabolism a bit and helps you to burn the calories taken in at the meal even faster.

DEVISING A "SELF-PLAN"

A technique for boosting motivation involves the writing of a self-plan. Our feeling of motivation can often be analyzed into two components: having goals and getting rewards for our achievements. Writing a plan helps us set our goals and reward our successes.

Increasing physical activity is an area of behavior in which many students report motivation problems. Write your overall goal at the top of a sheet of paper. (See example following.) In this case, it would be a goal to be achieved over a period of two weeks: "Increase my energy output to a total of 200 extra calories per day." Beneath that, write the specific ways to reach the goal: "Increasing my walking to an extra hour each day," or "Playing tennis for an hour, three times a week."

Next, you should create a gradual plan for approaching the end goal, specifying the steps you will take to achieve it each day. On walking, for example, you might list the following steps:

> Monday, ask husband if he'll walk with me after dinner; Tuesday, take a fifteen-minute walk after lunch; Wednesday and Thursday, walk fifteen minutes after lunch and fifteen minutes after dinner. On Friday, walk fifteen minutes after lunch and fifteen minutes after dinner [note that you don't have to increase the goal every day; take it slowly]. On Saturday and Sunday, walk a half hour after lunch or (on Sunday) after a late breakfast.

> In the second week, on Monday and Tuesday walk fifteen minutes after lunch and a half hour after dinner. On Wednesday and Thursday, again, fifteen minutes after lunch and a half hour after dinner. On Friday, walk a half hour after lunch and a half hour after dinner and finally, on the final weekend, walk an hour after lunch (or late Sunday breakfast).

This brings you up to nearly 200 calories (actually 180 for an hour of walking) per day in two weeks' time. Write these steps down on the left side of the page. Next to each step, leave a space to give yourself a check mark as credit for doing that step. You can count each check mark as a point and say that you have succeeded if you earn a certain number of points (for example, five out of seven). Or, you can give more possible points for each day; for example, a point for each fifteen minutes of walking.

The final part of the plan is crucial: There must be a reward for achievement. At the bottom of the sheet, write down a self-reward for completing the week successfully. It's important that the reward be readily available and that you not give it to yourself that week unless you achieved your goal (for example: going to the movies, or buying some item, or getting your hair done, or watching a favorite TV program, or going to the library, etc.). One client of ours used this system to motivate herself on physical activity by setting a goal of fifteen minutes an evening on her stationary bicycle (during TV commercial breaks). She used the method of one point per minute and gave herself money as a reward, dropping a nickel in a box for each minute, with a goal of five dollars to telephone her sister long-distance at the end of the week.

Work on this self-plan this week. The same technique can be used for other problems. It's important that you not see your self-plan as an "all or none" goal. Reward yourself for *each* step and know that you will have off days. If you miss a step, simply do it later or pick up where you left off as soon as you can.

This assignment includes a self-reward for a very important reason. Using a pleasure to reward yourself for some conscious program of change is a psychological principle that is often overlooked. Many people feel that self-rewards are somehow childish or even immoral. We hear people say, "I should do such-and-such just because it's right or good for me." Or, "Self-reward is a form of bribery." Perhaps it's true that ideally all activities should be inherently self-rewarding either because they are pleasurable or righteous. However, reality tells us that we need a boost to get into new things. If anything, we already rely heavily on rewards, but rewards from others—pats on the back from an outside judge. Self-reward lets us admit that we need reinforcement, but that we can take that power of judge and giver of pleasure onto ourselves.

SAMPLE SELF-PLAN FORM

Overall Goal: Increase my extra physical activity to 200 calories daily

Total Points Required: _12,24_

		2 Week Plan	Points for Each Step	
		Gradual Steps to Reach Goal	1st Day	2nd Day
WEEK 1	Monday Tuesday	Walk 15 minutes after lunch or dinner	1	1
	Wednesday Thursday	Walk 15 minutes after lunch and 15 minutes after dinner	2	2
	Friday	Walk 15 minutes after lunch and 15 minutes after dinner	2	
	Saturday Sunday	Walk 1/2 hour after lunch or after a late breakfast	2	2
		First Week Total - 12 points		
WEEK 2	Monday Tuesday	Walk 15 minutes after lunch and 1/2 hour after dinner	3	3
	Wednesday Thursday	Walk 15 minutes after lunch and 1/2 hour after dinner	3	3
	Friday	Walk 1/2 hour after lunch and 1/2 hour after dinner	4	4
	Saturday Sunday	Walk 1 hour after lunch or a late breakfast	4	4
		Second Week Total - 24 points		

Self-reward for successful completion of this self-plan:
Buy the new pair of shoes I've been wanting.

78

So each time you assign yourself a task to change your behavior, view it as a contract. Contracts have a payoff, and you deserve a reward written into the contract.

VICTORY LIST

At this point, it would be worthwhile to establish a victory record in a form that you can read regularly, much as you do the "Reasons to Lose Weight" card. Use a three-inch-by-five-inch card for this purpose. Write at the top the word "Victories." As you are aware of a major accomplishment, write it on the card. The list can include things directly related to eating, as well as other changes that you feel contribute to your self-control in eating. Read your Victory list frequently, especially before and after meals, but also at times when you feel discouraged about your progress. Here's a sample list of the type of victories you might include. You, of course, may have many that are not on this list. Notice that a victory may be a successful step along the way to a greater goal.

1. I eat more slowly and really taste my food.
2. My extra physical activity is up by 200 calories a day.
3. I take a walk most evenings after dinner.
4. My evenings are more active.
5. Predinner nibbling is under control four or more days a week.
6. I tell my husband when he sabotages me with tempting food.
7. I got my children to help out after dinner.
8. I can leave some food on my plate at some meals.

SUGGESTED PARTNER ACTIVITY

We would like you to consider the role of physical activity in your own life. Does your work require that you move a lot, or do you sit all day? Are physical activities enjoyable to you and a regular part of your leisure time? If so, who shares these activities with you? Do you play sports, hike, take walks? How would the amount of physical activity you engage in each day add up over a week's time in comparison to your partner's level of activity?

A good way for your partner to increase her enjoyment of exercise is to have company while she is doing it. She is devising her own personal plan for increasing her physical activity, and you should consider how to structure in some physically active recreation time together. Make a list of activities you could choose from together. At the least, we would like you to take a couple of brisk walks together this week. If you would rather do an alternate activity from your own list, that's fine.

Another way in which your partner can increase physical activity is to increase the amount of energy expended in regular everyday activities. Here are some things you can do with your partner that will help increase routine physical output: Park farther from your destination when you go out together, first in small amounts and then gradually increasing the distance. Use stairways instead of elevators. Don't use shortcuts when walking. If you ride the bus or are getting a ride, get yourselves dropped off a few blocks from where you're going. It may seem awkward to do these things at first, but eventually they become automatic. Remember, if your partner spends one hundred calories per day above the average output, without increasing eating, she should lose about ten extra pounds this year.

The effort that your partner makes to increase activity is a significant one. Notice and reinforce this effort.

chapter seven
REDUCING STRESS WITHOUT EATING

Stress affects us in two ways. First, there are the obvious big events in our lives: death or illness of a loved one, our own illness, changing residence, changing jobs, a distressing relationship, ending a relationship, getting married, having a child. This list intentionally includes events that we often consider positive. There is a lot of research to indicate that major life change, no matter how positive, produces a certain amount of stress. The second type of stress involves the tensions produced by daily living—everything from driving the freeway, to waiting in lines, to all of the irritations of various interactions with people. Hurrying, time pressure, the pressure to get work completed, minor scares, leaky faucets, and busy telephones all contribute to a more or less constant background level of stress. This is experienced as bodily tension of various sorts, a general feeling of discomfort or anxiety, or as fatigue.

We all have techniques to use when tension builds up: pacing, biting nails, smoking cigarettes, prayer or meditation, muscle relaxation, deep breathing, chewing gum, eating, etc. You may find this list a strange mixture of "good" and "bad" activities. Whether a technique is effective or destructive may not be immediately obvious. Chewing gum (especially sugar-free!) may work very well for someone. Another person may chew packs of gum and get nothing more than a sore jaw and a thinner wallet. Each of us has to have such techniques, but it's important to evaluate them periodically, using what business people sometimes call a cost/benefit analysis; that is, trying to weigh the cost (in finances, effort, physical damage, etc.) against the benefit in relief of tension. Also, in such an evaluation you must consider the possibility that a technique works too well and keeps you from directly solving a problem. Sometimes this possibility is a hard one to face—for example, recognizing that you are so effective in your meditation that you can calm your anger and avoid being assertive toward someone who is repeatedly infringing on your rights.

Regardless of the difficulty in periodically reevaluating your stress-reducing techniques, they are still an important part of everyone's life skills. Your interest in this program undoubtedly means that you have evaluated eating as a tension-reducing technique to be too costly for you in terms of the negative effects of being overweight. Take a look at the other techniques you use; compare them with those used by people around you. Is there a technique you think would be fairly effective, one which you would like to acquire or improve? Muscle relaxation is one we are focusing on in this chapter. It has a number of advantages, and you may want to include it more extensively in your bag of coping techniques. It can be fairly effective without being noticed by others, and has few, if any, negative side effects. The art in this technique is to focus on those muscles not needed for the main activity of the moment, and to relax as much of your body as you can, as much of the time as you can.

This relaxation skill will help you in several ways: First, as we have indicated, regular use can reduce the effect of stress, or unpleasure, in your life. This will be true whether you set aside regular times each day to relax all of your body or if you use differential relaxation (relaxing unused muscles) at various times that you feel tense. Second, the pleasurable effects of relaxation may increase your energy and ability to be involved in other pleasurable activities. Finally, muscle relaxation before and during meals (especially paired with the imagery techniques we will teach you later in this chapter) will reduce the tendency to eat in a hurried and compulsive way. All in all, relaxation is a skill that has great potential for reducing the mis-eating you do as a result of stress. Even more important, it is a skill that will help you lead the richer and more enjoyable life that will increase the chances of keeping off the weight you lose.

There are several ways to learn the relaxation technique. You can read through the following instructions and then practice, remembering as much as you can and improvising freely; you could have someone read them aloud to you; or you could read them aloud yourself, recording the instructions on a cassette. These instructions are also available on cassette from BMA Cassettes (200 Park Avenue South, New York, New York 10017), either as a single cassette or as part of our twelve-lecture series, *Comprehensive Weight Control*.

Now let's begin. Make sure you're wearing comfortable clothes and have thirty minutes or so of uninterrupted privacy. Leave a note on the door. Try to have the phone taken care of.

Take off your shoes. Sit in a comfortable chair. You're first going to relax your whole body by systematically tensing and releasing each of the major muscles.

1. Raise your feet a few inches off the floor, with your legs extended straight. Tense the muscles in your legs for a few moments. Hold the tension until your legs feel very heavy, then let go. You'll feel relaxation and warmth surge through your legs.

2. Tense your buttocks, as if you were trying to raise yourself off the seat of the chair. Hold the tension in your buttocks and then release it, sinking, comfortably relaxed, into the chair.

3. Pull in your stomach muscles. Hold the tension for a few moments and then relax.

4. Extend both arms in front of you, clench your fists and stiffen your arms. Imagine someone is pulling your arms, so that you feel the tension all the way across your back. Take a deep breath, expanding your chest. Hold it a few moments, then let go. Let your hands drop into your lap and feel the relaxation all through your body.

5. Scrunch the back of your neck down into your shoulders, then raise your shoulders, pulling the neck muscles tight. Hold it a few moments, then let go.

6. Squeeze your eyes shut, knit your brow, and clench your teeth so that you feel the tension all over your face. Hold it and then let go. Now all of the major muscles are relaxed. Close your eyes and just enjoy the feeling of warmth and relaxation.

Now let your imagination wander and think of a very pleasant location—the beach, a forest, an outdoor place you really enjoy. Try to imagine it as vividly as possible—the colors, the sounds, the feel of the air on your skin, even the pleasant smells. Spend a few moments concentrating on this scene. Don't worry if it comes and goes or your mind wanders. Just relax and enjoy the time.

Next imagine yourself walking in this favorite setting—in a garden, on the beach, wherever it's beautiful. Imagine your body moving along a path or along the beach. You are watching the passing scene. Your arms are swinging. You feel light and full of energy. Your body is tingling and alive. As you walk faster, you can feel the fresh air filling your lungs and the warm, vigorous movement of your arms and legs. You have a light, joyous feeling and can even imagine the pounds melting away as you walk vigorously along. After walking this way for a while, you stop to rest in a particularly beautiful spot. Your body is even more relaxed, just pleasantly warm.

Later, as soon as it's convenient, actually go for a short walk. Walk vigorously for ten minutes, if you can. Then stop and rest. Notice the same feelings in your body as you imagined; the lightness in your arms as you swing along, the pleasure of breathing. Imagine those pounds melting away as you walk. Enjoy the slightly tired, warm, and relaxed feeling when you stop to rest.

Try to practice this sequence once a day: Relax, imagine, then walk.

Now let's try an imagery sequence specifically related to eating. This will help you increase your relaxation during eating and increase your ability to resist eating foods you choose not to eat, or eating too much food. First, we will deepen your relaxation using a technique a bit like hypnosis, but which does not involve putting you in a deep trance; it just suggests more and more relaxation.

Now place your hands in your lap. Find a target spot on either hand and focus on it. That's right . . . hands and body relaxed . . . looking directly at the target. Look steadily at the target; while staring at it, remember this sequence or listen to a tape of the suggested scene. In a minute or two, your eyes may start to get tired. When that happens, just let them close gently and keep them closed. In a little while begin to count from one to twenty. You will feel yourself going further and further into a deep, restful state of relaxation, but you will be able to imagine any scene without disturbing yourself. One—you are going to relax . . . Two—down, down, deeply relaxed . . . Three, four—more and more relaxed . . . Five, six, seven—you are sinking deeper and deeper. Nothing will disturb you. . . . You are becoming very, very relaxed and you are finding it easy to just listen or to remember. . . . Eight, nine, ten—halfway there . . . eleven, twelve, thirteen, fourteen, fifteen—although deeply relaxed, you remember and imagine clearly. You will always remember and imagine distinctly, no matter how relaxed you are. . . . Sixteen, seventeen, eighteen—very deep. Nothing will disturb you. . . . You are going to experience many things vividly and clearly. . . . Nineteen, twenty. Very deep! That's it. Remain very comfortably relaxed throughout the following imagery exercise.

Get a clear image of yourself as the thin person you are becoming. See yourself as trim and fit, as you want to be. Imagine that you are that person choosing to eat some of your favorite food. See the food clearly in front of you. . . . Now imagine taking a small bite. Picture the sensation of it on your teeth and lips. Notice your mouth watering. Feel the food on your tongue and cheeks. Move it around your mouth. Really enjoy it to its utmost. Now imagine choosing whether to eat another bite. Each bite is delicious and satisfying. You can feel yourself relaxing more and more, feeling really nice as you slowly eat, enjoying every sensation of chewing, swallowing, and feeling your stomach slowly fill up. You can feel slightly full without feeling stuffed. As you begin to feel this way, you know a sense of strength and control, aware that you have complete freedom to choose whether to eat each bite. There is no sense of sacrifice or longing. You have eaten exactly what you want, in a safe way, in an amount that you have carefully chosen. This fact gives you a sense of satisfaction and a surge of energy to tackle the problems that face you.

The next time you eat, go through the critical points of this exercise again, this time actually eating in a slow and sensual way. First, tense and relax all of your muscles. Then, with the food in front of you, you will stop and check how you are feeling. Examine yourself for hunger sensations. Begin to eat in the same slow, sensual way that you did in your imagination. Then take the first bite. Notice every taste sensation—on your lips, tongue, teeth, against your cheeks. Chew very slowly. Really enjoy. Feel the food going down your throat. Feel it filling your stomach. Stop and choose at each bite, checking on how your stomach feels and what is happening to any other feeling. As you begin to feel slightly full and feel a sense of pleasant relaxation, you can choose to stop.

After any imagery exercise, count slowly to yourself from five back to one. As you count, you will become more and more wide awake and alert, but your body will continue to feel very relaxed. Five . . . Four . . . You're starting to feel awake. . . . Three . . . More awake and alert. Stretch your arms . . . Two . . . When you feel like it, open your eyes. . . . One, you feel completely awake and refreshed.

As a final summary for this chapter, let's look at tension during eating itself, tension that reduces awareness and increases mis-eating. As you examined your eating over the past couple of weeks, you may have noticed different kinds of tension:

1. Concern over what to choose and how much to serve yourself.
2. Anxious anticipation of that first bite.
3. Physical tension as you eat.
4. Social tension with others at the table.
5. Worrying about other problems during the meal.
6. Feeling in a hurry about some activity after the meal.
7. Worrying about how much you're eating.

As in other areas, the first step in solving a problem is to analyze and describe it. If you have identified one of these types of tension in yourself, write it out as a problem to solve. List as many details as you have observed (e.g., when it occurs and when it doesn't, specifically how you feel it in your body, and any other special aspect to the worries). Then list some solutions—some strategies to reduce the tension. Finally, try a strategy and record whether it is effective. The strategies will vary. Here are a few possible solutions for various kinds of tension:

1. Do the physical relaxation and imagery exercise before the meal. Do differential relaxation during eating, paying attention to which unneeded muscles can be systematically more relaxed.

2. Know exactly how many calories you want to *spend* on this meal before you select your food.

3. If eating slowly is hard when you're feeling ravenous, take three or four quick and large bites; then stop, put your utensils down, relax, and start again slowly and with awareness.

4. Consider what assertion steps are necessary with people who are disturbing your meal. Refer to Chapter 15 for methods on assertion and to Chapter 14 for particular problems with family members. Television, types of conversation, arguing—all can increase tension level.

5. Set aside a few minutes *after* the meal to relax, take a walk, and/or to review your problems and upcoming activities, so that you can defer mealtime worrying to another time.

We have taught you a simple relaxation and imagery sequence in this chapter. Practice from memory or with a tape recording a couple of times a day for the next week. Before dinner is a good time. So is before going to sleep, especially if you have even mild insomnia. Reviewing the imagery about physical exercise and eating just before sleep can help implant that learning. After a week or so of practice, you should be practicing full relaxation without a tape at a regular time each day and relaxing unused muscles whenever you notice tension.

TAKING DRUGS TO RELAX

The consumption of relaxation drugs (transquilizers, alcohol, tobacco, marijuana, and other legal or illegal substances) is so great in recent years that it boggles the mind. We can't devote much space here to this issue, except to note a few points on the relationship between drugs and eating. Chapter 12 devotes a section to alcohol, in the context of discussing restaurants.

Marijuana is apparently an increasingly popular alternative to alcohol. First, it is lower in calories (essentially zero). However, this advantage is probably offset by its effect on appetite. Alcohol is a depressant. Though it may increase eating at first because it relaxes and clouds judgment, it doesn't directly stimulate appetite. (Serious alcoholics often become malnourished, but please don't consider taking this route to weight loss.) Marijuana does seem to directly stimulate appetite, as well as to cloud judgment. Again, the strategy to control is planning. Know how a given amount of the drug typically affects you. Plan for a certain amount of calorie consumption; even prepare the type and quantity of food you want.

It is true that smoking tobacco does depress appetite and that quitting often does lead to a *moderate* weight gain. But this is not a reason to take up what is recognized more and more as a dangerous habit. If you are a smoker (especially if it is a moderate habit and not yet noticeably affecting your health), it may be best to postpone quitting (if you're planning to) until your weight problem and eating control are well in hand. Trying to quit smoking and lose weight at the same time is probably an undue strain, even though a few people do better on such a total-push program.

Probably the most important negative aspect of smoking, as it relates to eating, is its "signal" function. That is, we tend to put habits together: a cigarette with a drink, a cigarette after dinner, a cigarette with certain snacks. Examine these combinations in your own life and try to break them. Enjoy smoking if that is your decision, but try not to let cigarettes and food be combined. One possible exception to this rule is the case where smoking signals the end of eating—lighting a cigarette prevents further eating at the end of a meal.

SUGGESTED PARTNER ACTIVITY

The area of focus in this chapter is relaxation. If you can, help your partner by reading the step-by-step instructions aloud to her as she does the exercise to relax. If you have a tape recorder, make a recording of the instructions that she can play any time. Have your partner read the instructions while you try doing the relaxation exercise. The two of you might want to alternate—one reading, the other relaxing. Anything else you might do together that is relaxing for both of you can be significant in reducing the tensions that make life less pleasant than it could be. Be involved with your partner in at least one deliberate relaxation activity this week.

The areas of relaxation and stress management are most important in the long run. The benefits to both of you in incorporating relaxation into your routine, if you do so, will include greater energy, productivity, health, and, when you get used to it, pleasure. There is no doubt that it is an effort in the beginning. However, the pleasures you will derive will reward your efforts.

chapter eight
COPING
WITH EMOTIONS

In this chapter we will begin to deal with start controls in situations where a primary issue is an emotion that leads to mis-eating.

First, let's define the word *emotion*. Technically, the word refers to a sensation in your body to which you give a name. Your body gets aroused by some event (either real or imagined) and your mind says, "I feel scared, or sad, or anxious, or happy, or angry, etc." If we could simply express our anger (or other emotion) *directly* each time something occurred to arouse us, the emotion would be released. Instead, for one reason or another we can't get angry directly at various people, so the emotion is kept going and is confused by our thoughts about that person. Or, the anger is kept inside and we experience other bodily sensations as a result (tension in various places). Then we often do something to relieve the tension, such as get irritable with other people or eat. By this time we may not even be aware of what made us angry or that we were angry at all. We feel a vague sensation of tension and a desire to eat, knowing that eating tends to cover up tension and make us feel better temporarily. Unfortunately, eating has its own bad consequences later, as we know. So, what can be done about this type of sequence?

The solutions involve several possibilities:

1. Dealing with the causes. This solution is important, but in large part lies outside the scope of this book. Each of us has various and often tangled human relationships that evoke emotions. Factors related to our childhood experiences further complicate these relationships and our reactions to them. As you go through this book, examining and working on various factors that lead to miseating, you may indeed discover and decide to change some of these causes of emotions. The change process itself may be temporarily upsetting. You may seek other sources of education or counseling, or you may decide to try other strategies to live with situations such as those involving marital problems, problems in raising children, problems in asserting yourself, problems with your job, etc.

2. Becoming more perceptive about your emotions and what causes them, differentiating emotions from feelings of hunger.

3. Learning to express emotions more fully, or to relieve tensions without eating. This is an important approach which we will discuss briefly, but which again is difficult to teach in a book. We can give you suggestions that may help, but you may have to try other resources to expand your growth in this area.

Let us now discuss these topics in greater detail.

Recognizing Different Emotions

We will use the following exercise to improve the recognition of your emotions. Read through the following instructions and then try the exercise. You can also have someone read the instructions to you, or tape-record them and play back the tape to yourself.

Begin with the same relaxation exercise we taught you in Chapter 7.

Make sure you're wearing comfortable clothes and have 30 minutes or so of uninterrupted privacy. Take off your shoes. Sit in a comfortable chair. You're going to relax your whole body by systematically tensing and releasing each of the major muscles. Do these steps in order:

1. Raise your feet a few inches off the floor, with your legs extended straight. Tense the muscles in your legs for a few moments. Hold the tension until your legs feel very heavy, then let go. You'll feel relaxation and warmth surge through your legs.

2. Tense your buttocks, as if you were trying to raise yourself off the seat of the chair. Hold the tension in your buttocks and then release it, sinking, comfortably relaxed, into the chair.

3. Pull in your stomach muscles. Hold the tension for a few moments and then relax.

4. Extend both arms in front of you, clench your fists and stiffen your arms. Imagine someone is pulling your arms, so that you feel the tension all the way across your back. Take a deep breath, expanding your chest. Hold it a few moments, then let go. Let your hands drop into your lap and feel the relaxation all through your body.

5. Scrunch the back of your neck down into your shoulders, pulling the neck muscles tight. Hold it a few moments, then let go.

6. Squeeze your eyes shut, knit your brow, and clench your teeth so that you feel the tension all over your face. Hold it and then let go. Now all of the major muscles are relaxed. Close your eyes and just enjoy the feeling of warmth and relaxation.

Try to stay relaxed as much as possible. Remember the last time you felt upset by some situation. Think of the circumstances—where you were, the particular person you were with. Imagine the room as vividly as you can. Remember what happened, what was said, how you felt. Notice any sensations in your body now as you imagine this scene—muscle tension, perhaps tears, dryness in the mouth or throat—anything at all, no matter how small. Try to put one clear label on these sensations: "I felt angry," "I felt sad," "I felt scared"—whatever seems the clearest emotion.

Review in your mind the sensations of the emotion you felt and compare them mentally to the sensations of hunger you experienced when you did the slow-eating exercise after several hours of fasting. What are the differences, the similarities? Can you tell clearly the difference between this emotion and real hunger? Or are the sensations similar for you? Whether you are now more aware of differences or simply aware that you can be confused, you will be better able to ask yourself, the next time you feel a vague sensation that might lead you to eat, "Am I hungry, or is this some other emotion?" Finish the exercise by relaxing again and imagining that favorite pleasant scene (forest, beach, etc.).

During this week, as various events occur, notice the physical sensations of different emotions—anger, fear, joy, sexual frustration, sadness. Each time, compare how the emotions feel different or similar to the sensation of real hunger. As you recognize and feel your emotions, you will begin to know yourself better and develop a kind of catalog of your own sensations, so that you can begin to give a more accurate answer to the question, "Am I really hungry?"

Expressing Emotions and Relieving Tension

We cannot teach you how to express your anger more directly, or how to overcome all of your fears, or how to be more sexual. But we can give you some limited information and guidance in some of these areas.

ANGER. Anger is a very difficult emotion to cope with because there are many situations in which it's not safe to let the anger out directly, or in which you have decided it would be inappropriate to do so. Also, we have all—especially women—been taught in our society that shouting and getting loudly angry is just not acceptable. Whether this teaching is right or wrong, it's a fact of life. We can increase our expression of direct anger somewhat, and can get direct counseling for that purpose, but for most of us the leftover tensions from some unexpressed anger will be a common occurrence.

One way to deal with the tensions of unexpressed anger is to do regular release activities designed for the specific area of your body experiencing the tension. Do you get tense around the jaw, do your fists clench, is there tightness across the chest or in your legs? Which is your special pattern? The next time you notice unexpressed anger and its bodily sensation, try one of these release activities as soon afterward as you can:

1. Tension in the jaw—Take a small towel and hold it lightly with both hands. Put it in your mouth, as far back as you can without gagging. Bite down on it hard, pulling with your hands. Bite as hard as you can, feeling the tension in your jaw and the relief when you let go. As you bite, imagine the person and situation that made you angry most recently. Try this several times in succession.

2. Tension in the hands—Use the same towel, but for the hands, twist the towel as tightly as you can, again imagining the person and situation that recently made you angry. Notice the relief in your hands as you let go. Try it several times. Also, try making fists and punching your mattress as hard as you can.

3. Arms and neck—Find an old tennis racket, or buy a cheap one for this purpose. Stand next to a bed or couch with the racket held in both hands like a club. Raise it high over your head and whack the bed as hard as you can. Do this over and over again, until you're tired, imagining the person and situation that angered you. Notice the feeling of relaxation and relief when you stop.

4. Legs—Lie on a bed and kick your legs rhythmically, first one, then the other. Start slowly, then go faster. This is like a child's temper tantrum. Again, imagine the person and situation that angered you. Continue until tired, then relax and notice the feeling of relief.

5. Screaming and yelling—Each of the above exercises can be accompanied by screaming or yelling, if you have a place where this is possible. Or just screaming without the other body movements is very helpful. If you're worried about someone hearing you, scream into a pillow. Another good place to scream is in your car with the windows rolled up. Privately, yell obscenities at the person and situation that has angered you. Try these anger-expression exercises this week, to see which ones are helpful.

FEAR OR ANXIETY.   We can again only give you a few brief tips in this area.

1. Approach a feared situation in small steps, if possible. Plan a sequence of manageable steps to deal with a particular fear. Re-

hearse these in imagination or with a friend. For example, you might be afraid to ask your boss for a raise. Plan your strategy. Practice what you'll say with a friend, asking him to challenge your request the way the boss might. Rehearse together.

2. Use the relaxation exercise. When you feel anxious or tense, do all or part of the muscle tensing and relaxing sequence. Give yourself time each day to do a relaxation exercise.

LONELINESS.   Loneliness and inactivity are among the strongest stimulants for mis-eating. Do whatever you can to get out, join new groups, contact people. Any small start will be a great help. If you must be alone, spend as much of the time as possible out away from home and kitchen, even if your only plan is to go for a walk. Be aware of the most lonely times, and plan as much as possible to fill the void (which is really in your head and heart, not your stomach). We have many early childhood experiences associating closeness, especially to our mother, with being fed. It's possible to slip unconsciously into a pattern in which we feed ourselves as a way of recapturing that closeness we had (or wished for) as children.

BOREDOM.   This is not really an emotion. Some people confuse other emotions and say "I'm bored" when they're really lonely or scared and unable to get active. Examine your boredon carefully to see what's holding you back from new activities that involve being with people.

SEXUAL FRUSTRATION.   Dealing with sexual frustration is beyond the scope of this book. There are increasing numbers of books, courses, and counseling services geared to this problem. If it is an area of concern for you, help is available.

FEELING EXCITED.   You may find that an unexpected bonus, a sudden good happening in your life, will lead you to want to eat. Try squealing with delight, jumping up and down, and calling a friend to tell the good news.

SUGGESTED PARTNER ACTIVITY

We all get into difficulties sometimes because of our emotions, whether it is by mis-eating or in some other way. There are two basic aspects of the question for you to consider. One has to do with how you react to your partner and her emotions. The other aspect involves your handling of your own emotions.

When you notice that your partner is in a strong emotional state (one that you have known to lead her to mis-eat, or possibly to function less well, or just to be miserable), how do you react? The first step in dealing with another person's emotionality is, of course, to recognize it. Whether or not there is anything else you might choose to do about it, it is always less disturbing to *know* what is affecting you, rather than to react strongly to someone without knowing what sparked that reaction in you. Whether or not we are aware of it, it is usually impossible for most of us not to react strongly to strong emotion in someone else, especially when that someone is your spouse.

This topic will be of more concern to some of you and less to others. If your partner mis-eats because of emotional upsets, and if you would like to be of help in stopping the process of emotional mis-eating, we can provide a few general guidelines for you.

1. *Recognizing an emotional upset.* Most of us have characteristic ways of handling our emotional upsets, and your partner has hers. You may notice mis-eating behaviors, but also she may become quiet and withdrawn, or else nervously talkative. With some, the signs are very open and obvious; with others, the signs are very subtle—a particular set to the mouth, an unwillingness to let you catch her eyes. Tuning in to your own reactions can sometimes tip you off that something is going on in her. You may find yourself avoiding contact with her, you may notice that you're behaving in an overly concerned manner, or you may find anger or frustration rising in you. And of these can tip you off that she also is on edge.

2. *Helping her to express what is on her mind.* Once you have recognized her emotional upset, one way to help is to provide a listening ear. In general, there's not much you can do to solve her problems for her—many spouses get in trouble trying. If you can ask

her what's going on and simply hear her and acknowledge her difficulties, you are doing a lot to help her feel less alone with her problems.

3. *Dealing with your own apprehension about approaching her.* One of the reasons most of us will avoid someone who is upset is that we are afraid that he or she is upset with us personally. If that is the case, we fear being attacked, rejected, or made anxious by the one we are avoiding. The problem in avoiding someone who is emotional is that we don't find out where their upset is coming from. A typical scenario is one where the wife seems upset and her husband is afraid she is upset with him. Actually, she's upset with herself, or the kids, or a friend, or her mother. But many husbands never find this out. The husband might avoid her, get defensive or critical—and all because he is sure she is angry with him. She then actually *does* become angry at his behavior; then he may indeed be attacked, just as he feared. If he had known she wasn't angry at him in the first place, he might not have acted in the way that provoked her attack. The moral is, you may be better off finding out what is really up.

Another common reason for avoiding emotionality in another person is the feeling that you should be able to successfully remedy the problem for her. Some people just characteristically feel bad about themselves when their attempts to provide solutions are rejected by others; or, if tried, are then not successful. If this seems to fit for you, you are probably taking too much of a burden on yourself when you approach your partner and her upsets. If you have taken on this kind of responsibility for someone else, it is no wonder that sometimes you'd rather not be involved; it is no fun feeling like a failure time after time. If you could convince yourself that probably the *best* you can do for your partner is to keep her company and provide contact, so that she doesn't feel isolated with her feelings, then you will have gotten rid of your own heavy load *and* helped her out.

The second issue is how you handle your own emotions. Your partner has received suggestions for releasing problem emotions which you might also find useful for yourself. As far as miseating is concerned, how you handle your emotions also affects your spouse. If you come home from work tense or irritable with others, you might mis-eat—and provide a poor model for your partner. Or you might be edgy with her and cause tension that might lead her to mis-eat. Recognizing your own feelings and sharing them with each other can provide a more open, responsive relationship.

chapter nine
DOUBLE YOUR PLEASURE AND FIGHT DEPRESSION

It is generally important for permanent weight control to increase pleasure in your life. Being aware of what gives you pleasure has two important functions in permanent weight control: You will be able to make substitutes for eating and reward yourself for change.

First, you have to face the fact that eating is pleasurable and that depriving yourself of part of that pleasure leaves a gap. No matter how successful you are in slowing down the eating process and making it more sensuous and pleasurable, the quick, almost druglike jolts of pleasure from food, especially from things like cookies and candy, have to be less frequent if your weight is to be managed. So you have to find replacements, if possible. Feed your body in other ways; stimulate your mind; nourish your soul.

It's amazing how we can go for so long without experiencing any other pleasure than flopping in front of a television set, going to sleep, or, of course, eating. We know there is a lot for us out there, but we remain in a kind of apathetic fog, too passive to try something new or even to go back to an old pleasure that was once easy.

As with many of the other things we're teaching you in this book, increasing your pleasure may call for sharpened awareness and structure. We would like to help you with this, but are aware of a kind of natural resistance people have to being advised to "go out and enjoy life." When you're feeling low, that kind of advice can easily drive you further back into your shell. However, this area is so important we feel that we have to gently prod you and hope that you'll take a step or two. Once you begin to do something pleasurable, you can get hooked and develop what one author called a "positive addiction."

We have included several forms to help you become more aware of possible pleasures and help you structure your effort to try some things. The first is entitled "My Everyday Checklist of Pleasures." This is a list of about fifty activities that many people describe as pleasurable, and which are generally available without great cost or effort. We think you'll be surprised at some of the things on the list—because they're so simple and obvious. You probably do many of them and don't attend to how pleasurable they are or that they are acts you can consciously choose to do when you feel in the need of a pick-me-up. Take a few moments to look over the list now.

Can you add to the list? Check those you want to do more often. For the next week, consciously make an effort to increase the frequency of these activities. Plan your days so that at key times you make room for one of these activities, and then make a conscious effort to do it.

By now your diaries will have given you a clearer picture of the times during the day or week or month when you are most vulnerable to mis-eating. The pleasure list can be your best weapon at these times. You might find it a bit strange to be instructed to enjoy yourself, but go ahead anyway. Most people see weight control as a horrendous act of will. We feel that the little things you do to be nice to yourself will make eating less food not so difficult to bear.

The second form on pleasure is entitled "My Special Pleasures List." These are bigger—they take more effort or cost more. We made the separation for two reasons: first, to emphasize the simplicity and ease of the items on the first list; second, to introduce you to the use of pleasures as self-rewards, which we discuss in the next section. Make copies of both forms and fill them out for the next two weeks. If it's a helpful assignment, you can continue it longer. After a week or two of experience, you should be able to make a briefer list of pleasures that are available for use. Write this list on a three-inch-by-five-inch card, and carry it in your wallet or purse. Or, you can use an item as a reward after completing some exercise or new behavior or achieving a victory over temptation.

Often the experience of pleasure is a combination of familiarity and newness. New activities can be a bit scary. Until we become comfortable enough with them, that fear may be just enough to stop us from doing them. As a result, we rely on the familiar to the point that it becomes boring. Somewhere in between is a level of flexibility that will allow you to try new things and still enjoy the comfort of those broken-in shoes. The third form in this chapter is entitled "Flexibility Inventory."

We would like you to take another step in the direction of flexibility with regard to eating-related habits. First, take an inventory of areas where you may be a victim of habit. The Flexibility Inventory sheet lists a number of topics for self-examination. For each one, briefly describe any habits you have. As an example, under Breakfast you might say, "Never eat breakfast," or "Always have toast and coffee."

Each topic is designed simply as a stimulus to help you recognize various ways you tend to live by habit. You can add any others you think are interesting for you. These habits aren't necessarily either good or bad. We are aiming for awareness, choice, and flexibility. By becoming aware of your choices and intentionally going against a habit for a while, you not only broaden your possibilities in that area of your life, but you build up the attitude of flexibility. This attitude says, in effect, "I can change if I want to. These are always possibilities. I am in control. I need never be bored or stuck."

It's one thing to recognize habits and alternatives, but quite another to actually do new things and feel the flexibility that is a possibility.

To help you do this, we would like you to develop a definite self-plan and some form of self-reward for trying this experiment. On the back of the Flexibility Inventory is a plan sheet designed for two weeks. For each week, list at least three areas in which you will try to break a habit and use new responses you listed on the inventory. At the bottom of the sheet is a space to list what your self-reward will be, (e.g., "I'll go to a movie Saturday night if I get at least fifteen checks on the plan sheet").

A word of caution about this plan: Don't be too serious about it. It is not intended necessarily to solve important problems. We simply want you to try new things. They can be silly, fun ways to change your routine. You may even decide you like all of your old habits better. That's fine. Again, the important thing is to build up the flexibility attitude—it can be fun to experiment.

EMPHASIZING PLEASURE AS SELF-REWARD

As you know by now, weight loss is often not a predictable, regular process. You can work very hard for several days and not see any results, then suddenly lose a pound. At best, there is a delay of a day before you see results on the scale. If you are going to achieve permanent control, you have to develop a wide range of skills (from eating awareness to increased activity to more assertiveness, and so on). If any skill is to improve, you must reinforce it. Some behaviors have built-in rewards. For example, if you take up a sport, you often get hooked on the satisfaction of playing and seeing yourself improve. But others are not as directly rewarding (e.g., leaving food on your plate). To some extent these can be reinforced by complimenting yourself ("I did it!" "I'm improving," "I've mastered that," etc.), or by the act of rating yourself and seeing the ratings increase. However, a concrete reward can be very effective. After all, you wouldn't work just for the praise of your employer. So don't be embarrassed about being your own boss and paying off for production of good work. In fact, the more you are your own boss the better you'll feel.

A client told us of her very effective reward system. Every day that she stays under her daily calorie goal, she put one dollar in a special piggy bank. She was saving up for an expensive handbag she had seen and wanted. Your particular splurge can be anything from a special purchase to an evening on the town.

One important kind of self-reward is the simple reminder of a job well done. This is a good point, to repeat an idea we described in Chapter 6. Keep a Victory List. At times when things look bleak, it's good to remind yourself of how much you've accomplished. But also, the act of adding to the list and reading it over is an excellent self-reward for completing an assignment, resisting a temptation, or making any advance in your efforts to change.

A couple of final thoughts on stimulating yourself to try new, pleasurable activities. First, look for trade-offs with friends. Often, you can find someone who's already into tennis, embroidery, or whatever the activity. He or she would be delighted to help you start; in return, you can help them to begin an activity you're already comfortable with.

A PLEASURABLE EVENING

Finally, here's a technique to give yourself that little extra push to do something you think might be pleasurable but which for some reason you're resisting (fear, embarrassment, apathy?). Let's say you have an evening with no important obligations and you'd like to do something nice and avoid sitting in front of the TV. List six things you could do, and number them. They may vary in cost and desirability, but all are *possible* and all might be pleasurable if you tried them. Then agree with yourself to choose an activity for the evening by chance. Roll a die from a pair of dice, and do the activity you listed for the number (one to six) that comes up.

You may feel that it is childish or somehow passive to let chance decide for you. But remember, *you* are listing the choices and *you* are committing yourself to do one of those activities. And that may be more active and adult than sitting in front of the TV. Once you roll the die, you will face an important moment of hesitation. "Can I do that?" "Do I really want to?" You must agree to follow the die and push yourself past that hesitation. Once into an activity, you have a good chance of enjoying yourself. The next time you may be more certain of what you want to do and not have to use dice. Or, you may find this an enjoyable way to get yourself into activities that interest you but which you rarely give yourself the opportunity to enjoy.

DEPRESSION AND PLEASURE

Psychologists have various theories about the causes of depression, ranging from biochemical imbalance to grief over loss of love. Whatever the cause, it seems clear that the experience of depression has two common features: 1) negative self-evaluation or criticism ("I'm a failure," "I'm no good," etc.) and 2) reduced levels of experiencing pleasure. While serious depression is often associated with loss of appetite, moderate depression may well lead to overeating and underactivity, with subsequent weight gain. This chapter, along with the chapter on physical activity and relaxation, gives you an antidote to both features of depression. Self-reward for making changes and conscious effort to increase pleasure in your life may be the best method to ward off depression.

SUGGESTED PARTNER ACTIVITIES

The suggestion for this chapter is simple and straightforward—join your partner in increasing pleasure in her life. Try sitting down together and writing out a "Mutual Pleasures" list. Include things you now enjoy, have enjoyed in the past, or even might enjoy in the future. You can draw on the list either to directly reward something you've achieved together or to find ideas to counteract times when one or both of you feel down.

MY EVERYDAY CHECKLIST OF PLEASURES

ITEM	WANT TO DO THIS MORE (✓)	DID TODAY?			ENJOYMENT Rate 1 - 5
		A lot	Some	None	
1. Walking or sitting in the sun					
2. Wearing my favorite clothes					
3. Seeing and hearing the sights and sounds of nature					
4. Noticing something I've never seen before					
5. Enjoying the luxury of a quiet time					
6. Being with people I like					
7. Giving myself a manicure and/or pedicure					
8. Seeing an old friend					
9. Offering my help or advice					
10. Having a frank and open discussion					
11. Being with someone I love					
12. Making love					
13. Meeting someone new					
14. Playing with or just being with animals					
15. Listening to music					
16. Thinking about something good in the future					
17. Resting after strenuous effort					
18. Stretching and then relaxing all my muscles					
19. Dancing					
20. Singing or humming					
21. Working on my hobby					
22. Making spare time for myself					
23. Reading a favorite magazine					
24. Reading poetry, a book, or a play					
25. Learning to do something new					
26. Planning or organizing something					
27. Watching a favorite TV program					
28. Planning a vacation or a trip -- or just a day off					
29. Doing a job well					

ITEM	WANT TO DO THIS MORE (✓)	DID TODAY? A lot	Some	None	ENJOYMENT Rate 1 - 5
30. Going to a restaurant, play, or movie					
31. Listening to the radio					
32. Relaxing with a cup of coffee or tea					
33. Making someone feel good					
34. Solving a personal problem					
35. Taking a nap					
36. Watching a sunrise or a sunset					
37. Caring for a plant or animal					
38. Laughing with people					
39. Touching and being close to someone I like or love					
40. Telling someone about what I've said or done					
41. Eating good food and enjoying every bite					
42. Doing a project my own way					
43. Taking a bath or shower					
44. Taking the time to look better than usual					
45. Feeling sexually attractive					
46. The nice feeling of crisp fresh sheets on my bed					
47. Brushing my hair and massaging my scalp					
48. Washing my hair with a fresh smelling shampoo					
49. Doing something I didn't think I could do					
50. Smoothing on hand lotion or a body cream or oil					
51. Feeling the fresh taste in my mouth after I brush my teeth					
52. Wearing a splash of cologne, after-shave, or perfume					
53. Asking someone to scratch my back or give me a good neck rub					

MY SPECIAL PLEASURES LIST

Special treats I want to have more often (or begin to have)
because I deserve them and because I want to enjoy myself more)

ITEM	Check (✓) if item appeals to me	When do I plan to do it? This week? month? year?	Date(s) I actually engage in this
1. BUY MYSELF SOMETHING FRIVOLOUS AS A PRESENT TO MYSELF, such as:			
a. Literally, give myself a bouquet -- even if it's just from the grocery store (plant or cut flowers)			
b. Buy myself an expensive magazine.			
c. Get a new wallet or keychain before I really need it			
d. A nonessential toiletry or cosmetic such as an expensive lipstick, soap, or makeup; a hot-lather shave; or a small personal appliance (curling iron, tennis-ball revitalizer, etc.)			
2. INDULGE MYSELF PHYSICALLY IN SOME "OUT-LANDISH" WAY, such as:			
a. Pour myself a bubble bath, sprinkle the water with flower petals, and sit in the tub and relax while I read a new magazine and play a favorite record			
b. Splurge on a professional facial, manicure, or pedicure. (or give myself the works)			
c. Have a hot-oil scalp treatment or go to a hairdresser for a good shampoo			
d. Get myself a massage			
e. Spend a day or a week or whatever at a spa or health club--or go visit one to see about joining later even if I can't afford it now			
3. FIX UP SOMETHING OLD SO I CAN USE IT NOW:			
a. Get a favorite purse, comfortable pair of shoes, or an appliance repaired			
b. Get a tennis racket restrung or a musical instrument tuned or repaired			

MY SPECIAL PLEASURES LIST - continued	Items that appeal	When do I plan to do it? This week? month? year?	Date(s) I actually engage in this
4. BUY MYSELF JUST ONE OF SOME ITEM THAT NORMALLY COMES IN SETS AND RESERVE THAT ONE ITEM JUST FOR ME:			
a. One beautiful china cup & saucer			
b. Just one rose for my table, my desk at work, my bathroom, or my bedroom			
c. One bathroom accessory that appeals to me most out of a group of things such as a fancy soap dish or hand lotion dispenser			
5. MAKE A ROUTINE EVENT SPECIAL:			
a. Use candles, flowers, and cloth napkins at dinner			
b. Plan something I want to see or do particularly on a daily walk			
c. Plan something new to do tonight just before I go to bed			
d. Drink my usual juice out of a wine glass or put a doily under my teacup			
e. Next time I wash my car, I'll get the dashboard polished or buy a good-smelling car air freshener.			
f. Get a new organizer tray for cosmetics, bath, or desk			
6. MAKE A POINT OF SEEING OR DOING SOMETHING I'VE WANTED TO DO FOR A LONG TIME BUT HAVE NEVER GOTTEN AROUND TO:			
a. Get a season pass to a sport I enjoy			
b. Go to some local attraction, museum, club, movie, or play that I've always planned to go to			
c. Make a start at a hobby I've thought about for years			
d. Get my ears pierced or go to the podiatrist about my feet			
7. CONTACT A FRIEND I HAVEN'T SEEN FOR YEARS			
8. MY OWN ITEMS (continued on next page)			
a.			
b.			

WEIGHT REDUCTION

Flexibility Inventory

	Topic	What I do now	New things I could do
1.	Breakfast		
2.	Foods I eat every day		
3.	Food I never eat		
4.	Time I eat dinner		
5.	Foods I always eat together (e.g., meat and potatoes)		
6.	The order in which I eat my meal (e.g., dessert is always last)		
7.	What I do right after dinner		
8.	What I do as soon as I get home from work (or most of a day off)		
9.	What I do on my lunch hour (or right after lunch)		
10.	(List at least one more of your own)		

FLEXIBILITY PLAN SHEET

First Week

Habit to be broken or new activity	Mon.	Tues.	Wed.	Thurs.	Fri.	Sat.	Sun.
1.							
2.							
3.							

Self-reward (list reward and how many days checked off are required for the reward):

_____

Second Week

Habit to be broken or new activity	Mon.	Tues.	Wed.	Thurs.	Fri.	Sat.	Sun.
1.							
2.							
3.							

Self-reward (list reward and how many days checked off are required for the reward):

_____

VICTORIES

1. I gave my 5-lb. box of Valentine chocolates to a skinny friend.
2. I am jogging 3 times a week — regularly!
3. I am no longer a member in the "Clean Plate Club."
4. I'm spending only meal preparation time in the kitchen.

chapter ten
"I'M A TRAVELING MAN"

Chapter 9 discussed the importance of increasing pleasure in your life. The more you are able and willing to give yourself pleasure in ways other than eating, the less you will be stimulated to eat as a way to produce pleasure. We have emphasized the principle that the more pleasurable eating is in itself, the less quantity you should have to consume. If you are eating in a relaxed, aware way, each mouthful will give you more pleasure.

A vacation is an ideal time to explore the meaning of pleasure for yourself. According to the dictionary, the word *vacation* has two kinds of meanings: 1) a time of freedom from work, and 2) a time of recreation. What does freedom from work mean to you? What do you need a rest *from*, an escape *from*? The whole idea here seems to be that there is something about our everyday lives that is *un*-pleasurable. Therefore, we periodically earn a release: *free* time. Unfortunately, this is the state of affairs for most of us, whether we work for someone else, or for our customers, or for our family.

There are craftsmen, artists, and even some people in routine jobs who seem to get a great deal of pleasure from their work and/or from the people they work with. Various sociological studies and our own observations lead us to conclude that these people are in the minority. It seems likely that many of you do not find your daily routine pleasurable. Some might even argue that this is a major reason for mis-eating.

There is another aspect of the freedom part of the definition of vacation. Our daily routine, its stress and its boredom, is intimately tied to our relationships with those people who are close to us. We spend fairly regular times with our spouse, children, friends, relatives—times governed by our work schedule and the schedules of others. Furthermore, our mood and the amount of energy we have when we are with those people are affected by the daily stresses of work routine. So, to some extent, the *un*pleasure of work spills over into the limited times when we could be having pleasure with those around us.

We can see then that a vacation is an escape *from* unpleasure, hopefully *to* pleasure. If you're like most of us, your vacation time is precious and limited; you want to plan to get the most out of it—the most escape and the most pleasure. If there ever was a time to be selfish, this is it. *Creative selfishness* allows you to provide for the desires of those around you in a way that maximizes your own pleasure. Every parent knows this principle; it's called "Finding a babysitter the kids enjoy being with."

The kind of examination of the meaning of vacations we have been doing has practical implications. We are suggesting that you plan your vacation by taking several definite steps:

1. Examine what about your daily routine you want to escape from. For example, if your routine is a hectic, crammed schedule, it's vital that you not repeat this pattern on your vacation. There's an expression, "Taking a busman's holiday." Many people do this literally. They do a lot of strenuous driving daily, then spend their vacation driving. That's fine if it's what you want, but be aware of the choice.

2. Consider carefully the kind of pleasure and freedom you are escaping to. Here's the extension of what we have been harping on about pleasure. A vacation is a time to consider what you like to do most. It may be a very active time or it may be staying home with the time to enjoy whatever, at your leisure. Your vacation will be most successful if you find ways to give yourself pleasures that carry over to nonvacation life—a hobby, the enjoyment of walking, time alone, time with your spouse.

3. Hold a family conference. Some of us vacation alone, but most of us have some arranging to do with family and friends.

Prior to a vacation is a good time to get the cooperation of those around you. Try to discuss openly the possibilities, the limitations, the conflicting needs. Then move on to specific planning, both to solve problems and to get the pleasure you're seeking. At this stage the planning itself will become pleasurable. A good vacation has a spread effect—from the pleasure of planning through to the glow of remembering. The negative aspects also spread. You may get tense in advance and be frustrated and angry afterward. Part of your conference can be a review of the last vacation. What did you like the best? What were the problems?

What does all of this have to do with eating and weight control? The main thing, of course, is our contention that eating is a way of giving ourselves pleasure. When we are lacking pleasure in other activities, we mis-eat.

The other side of the coin is the association of eating *with* pleasure. When we are having pleasure, we believe that eating will make that pleasurable time even better. A vacation is often a time when both of these principles are exaggerated. However, it also is a time when you can attend to giving yourself more pleasure in noneating ways, as well as attending to ways that you can enjoy eating while still limiting the quantities you eat. It's important to emphasize that a vacation can lead to an increase in eating for two opposing reasons: (1) You relax and let down control, and/or (2) You get tense and eat to relieve the added tension. Obviously, the strategy you use to control your eating will depend on which of these two reasons is more important at any given time.

HERE ARE SEVEN BASIC PRINCIPLES

1. It's okay to let down control on a vacation, but always look for compromises between strict control and complete abandon. Plan to *maintain* your weight; don't worry about not *losing* weight. Try to figure a daily calorie goal that will achieve temporary maintenance.

2. Try to do as much diary keeping as possible. Do some of the self-control exercises covered in this program, but don't push yourself; eat with awareness as much as possible.

3. If you tend to be tense on a vacation, a careful analysis in advance is really important. A vacation is supposed to be enjoyable. If yours tends not to be, then ask why and what you can do about it. This may be an important area for new assertiveness, to get the kind of vacation *you* really want. Getting what you want extends into the vacation itself. Beware of extended periods when you are doing what others want and not what you like. This kind of frustration often leads to mis-eating.

4. Plan daily times to relax; try not to get overtired. Jet lag on long trips is often a problem. Be aware of how time-zone changes tire you and throw off your eating rhythms, as well as sleep.

5. If you haven't read the chapter on restaurant eating (Chapter 12) before you go on vacation, it would be a good idea to cover it, because restaurants are such an intimate part of travel. Chapter 12 will also help you to be especially careful about alcohol during your vacation.

6. Try to balance rest with activity. Look for enjoyable ways to be active. If you can keep moderate control of the special eating temptations, the extra activity will often compensate. While you want to get enough sleep, beware of excessive sleep during vacations. This cuts down your energy output and sometimes increases eating.

7. Beware of reentry problems. Coming back from a vacation is often a letdown. Review your weight situation and plan necessary recovery strategies, but also plan for some extra pleasures to offset post-vacation blues. Try to get gradually back to regular activities. Sometimes it's valuable to allow an easy day at home before getting back to work, full steam.

Here are a few additional points of interest:

1. Visiting relatives, especially parents, who haven't seen you in a while can be a difficult problem. You will have to make some advance decisions about how and when you will want to be assertive about food. You'll also need an advance decision about what you'll say about your weight and diet, if anything (your right to remain silent is guaranteed by the Constitution). If you're traveling

with your spouse, discussing a common strategy to handle the relatives will be helpful.

2. Weigh yourself frequently, but remember that scales vary widely. Use the weighing more as a reminder than as an accurate measure of your real weight.

3. Being cooped up in a car is very likely to lead you to eat. Arrange regular breaks and physical activity. Carry along some relatively low-calorie snacks (labeled as to calorie value), but try a self-contract that says, "No eating while the car is in motion." When you stop for a rest, use your own snack food, and try for a ten-minute walk. Using low-calorie liquids during driving will also help. Finally, discuss the problem with your car mates and get their cooperation. Being cooped up in a plane, where food and alcohol are plentiful, is an even greater challenge. Walking seems to be important, both to control boredom and reduce the effects of jet lag. So, this is a good situation in which to remind yourself to keep your body in motion.

chapter eleven
DOWNFALL FOODS AND HARD TIMES: 'TIS THE SEASON TO BE JOLLY

Our chapters on start and stop controls have not yet dealt with a difficult issue: how to handle certain high-calorie, high-temptation foods. Each of us has these favorite foods. Usually, they are sweets or other high-calorie foods. If there are people with cravings for lettuce, they must be fairly rare (or very secretive)!

The underlying philosophy of this program is that we should aim for sufficient self-control to enjoy all foods in moderation. This differs from the view that some people are "foodaholics"—allergic and addicted to certain high-carbohydrate foods. The foodaholic must aim for total abstention from such foods; otherwise, he or she will suffer from a form of blackout and binge similar to that reported by alcoholics. We believe, to the contrary, that most overweight people *can* work toward controlled eating of all foods.

In any case, each of you can determine for yourself whether you can achieve the level of self-control necessary to eat *some* candy, *some* cake, *some* ice cream, or *some* of any food that has been a severe problem for you.

You may decide that for health reasons, or any other reason, that you won't eat candy ever again. That's fine, if this is a comfortable decision for you. Then your self-control tasks for these foods are entirely start controls—that is, learning to say no to these foods, avoiding temptations, finding substitute foods and activities, and so forth.

117

But for many people total abstinence is not a permanent solution. Sooner or later you may reach a point of deciding that you can stand it no longer. Unfortunately, what might happen is a colossal binge of proportions that satisfy the tension of the long period of deprivation.

It is not possible within the scope of this program to give you a simple step-by-step formula that will guarantee you strength and control of all high-temptation foods in all possible situations.

Even so, we can give you guidelines and a positive approach and view of the problem. The most important message is that the control of dangerous foods is not a "black or white" situation. Foods are not either always safe and controllable or dangerous and addictive. Unlike the case for the severe alcoholic, you can experiment with controlled eating of these foods without doing yourself severe damage.

Reintroducing a high-temptation food must be done with preparation and knowledge. You must ask yourself questions, such as:

1. Do I want to reintroduce this food back into my diet? What size portion can I afford in my calorie allowance?
2. Do I feel comfortable enough with my self-control skills (especially stopping) to try a gradual reintroduction at this time?
3. Do I have a lot of craving for this food? Has the tension of this craving built up in the past and led to a serious binge?
4. Does the dangerousness of this food change from time to time or situation to situation? That is, can I control myself, for example, early in the day with someone else present but not dare touch it alone at night?

We have stated that foods are not all black or all white, controllable or untouchable. Here are two principles:

Some of your dangerously tempting foods are slightly less dangerous than others.

A high-calorie temptation food may be controllable at certain times and places but deadly in other situations or times of day.

Observe yourself or try remembering what foods and situations are difficult for you. When mis-eating occurs, notice the time, place, and food involved.

The first step is awareness. Don't expect to come up with a list all in one week, or even one month. Just keep your eyes open and watch yourself. Are you most tempted at lunch with a friend over a dessert menu? Or is it alone at 2 A.M.?

Having information that is specific (How dangerous is the food? When is it most dangerous?) is the first step and probably the most important one.

The key toward solving a self-control problem is to take it in very small steps. We don't want you to jump in and decide to tackle the toughest, most dangerous food in your life first. We also don't want you to decide all at once to conquer your most vulnerable situation (for example, 2 A.M. refrigerator raiding) just because your husband is going on a business trip this week and you'll be alone.

Conquering dangerous foods is the most difficult step you will ever have to take in weight control. It won't be done in a few weeks or even a few months. You are battling lifetime habits against tremendous odds. You will have some successes and some setbacks. Oddly enough, research has shown that people who have a few setbacks and pick themselves up, take one step backward, and start again are the most successful—more successful than those with a "perfect record." You might say that those who were *always* perfectly successful during their practice runs were devastated and felt total failure when one slip or one binge occurred in a subsequent situation. When a setback occurs for you, the message is "I took too large a step," *not* "I'll never be able to eat this food." Gradualness is the key. Give yourself as many practice tries as you need to master a food.

There are a few rules to keep in mind:

1. At first, keep a limited supply of the food around, to protect yourself. As you become comfortable with your stopping ability with this food, you can have more of it available.

2. Don't decide to take on the challenge if you're feeling low,

tired, unhappy, lonely, irritable, or just bad in general. Choose a time when you feel strong and good about yourself.

3. Go in very small steps. Don't decide to practice a more dangerous situation just because the opportunity arises. Stay with each stage repeatedly until you feel confident, before trying something more tempting.

4. When you are eating, eat slowly and really attend to all of the taste sensations in the food.

5. When you are working step by step on controlling a particular tempting food, don't feel the need to demonstrate your capability every chance you get. Even though you feel you can control potato chips at a party, don't "test yourself" at every party. Go with how you feel at the time and whether you really want the food at that particular party. Also, consider whether you really want to spend the calories.

For the coming weeks, observe yourself and think about whether you want to gradually reintroduce highly tempting foods. For the present time, analyze which foods and which situations are the most difficult. It may be a long time before you actually decide to take the first small step toward this kind of self-control.

"'TIS THE SEASON TO BE JOLLY"

You may be in the midst of working on control of high-temptation foods when the highest temptation time of the year comes along.

Think of Thanksgiving and Christmas; what are your first thoughts or images? Almost everyone will have some picture involving food. Joyous occasions are always associated with good eating, and in our culture those of us with weight problems have come to expect to add pounds in the six weeks from Thanksgiving until after New Years Day. Why do we overeat especially at this time and what can we do to minimize the damage?

Some male chauvinist recently joked, "A woman's place is in the oven." Part of our sexist culture has exaggerated the importance of cooking as a woman's way of being accepted, admired, and loved. To be good at feeding a family is still, for many women, the primary route to self-esteem. The more traditional the family, the more this is true. And if the success in this role also leads the woman to be well fed and well rounded herself, this is often seen as a small price to pay by a husband who reaps the benefits of a nurturing wife who takes care of him and doesn't threaten his role by becoming a bread *winner* instead of a bread *baker*. Besides, he gets the added advantage of keeping her largely out of sight and out of trim so that she is less attractive to other men who tend to share the modern bias that slim equals attractive.

If the modern woman can accept her role and continue to have many satisfactions in her marriage, being overweight (unless it *leads* to medical complications) could be easily tolerated. But men, and other women, seldom can let the matter rest here, and instead proceed to place added pressure to lose weight and achieve or restore the much-valued slim figure. So, many women, whether married or not, must continually struggle to resolve this conflict, and they find the conflict especially difficult in the holiday season, when cooking and baking rich foods are so rewarded at the same time that parties and entertaining increase the pressure to be attractive.

There are other reasons why the holiday season is difficult for the weight-conscious, both women and men. The social and even religious stimuli for preparing special foods makes refusing food extremely difficult in social situations. If a hostess or a guest provides food, we feel great pressure not to offend. This is especially true if the giver has special importance for us—a boss or a parent, for example.

Eating has become almost inseparable from socializing. Gifts of food or drink are routinely expected. Food oils the machinery of socializing in situations where there is almost no other activity to occupy the guests. Conversation seems easier with food and drink in hand. If all else fails to enliven a dull interaction, you can always say, "Excuse me, I'm going to get another drink (or more food)."

As the religious and cultural traditions of the holidays become weaker, the desire increases to recapture the flavor of "Christmas past," especially to provide our children with the kind of memories we cherish. With increasing mobility, we are often separated from families; so that the memories seem to focus more and more on the material substance of the holidays—"visions of sugarplums danced through their heads."

Finally, there is another set of reasons for overeating during holidays, which center around the negative emotions evoked. Contact with normally distant relatives, especially parents, may produce conflict and anger that is difficult to resolve when we are supposed to be so loving and having a good time. Not to have contact exaggerates loneliness at this time of year, as we see others who seem to have so much more, especially in the fantasies presented on television. Our childhood may have been wonderful or terrible, but the resulting sadness is similar if we feel we can't possibly have what we want or need as adults. Whatever the negative emotions, we have the solution readily at hand, that ever-present tranquilizer and antidepressant: food.

WHAT CAN BE DONE?

What follows is an effort to apply the principles and techniques presented throughout this book to problems of the holiday season.

The first point that must be covered is the establishing of an overall goal for your weight during the holiday season. This will vary depending on where you may be in a weight-loss or maintenance program. But for everyone, a good principle is not to be too hard on yourself and to set *moderate* goals. It may be best to agree with yourself to try to maintain your weight and not attempt further loss at this difficult time. Achieving a more moderate goal will boost your motivation to take additional steps after the first of the new year.

As with so many of the problem-solving suggestions we have made, a primary concern is to use time to your advantage. Plan ahead to deal with problems rather than letting them catch you unprepared. Take the time and effort to write out a list of the specific problems you anticipate and the possible solutions that might work for you. When you construct such a self-plan, remember to be as concrete as you can about the steps you intend to take and to include some rewards for yourself for taking any of these steps. For example, keeping up your physical activity (sports, exercises, walking) may be part of your plan. Analyze how the holiday season will obstruct such activities; list ways to change your pattern and fit them in. You may routinely participate in some sport on Saturdays, but now have to give it up to do Christmas shopping. An hour of tennis singles roughly burns 300–400 calories. Could you plan an extra half hour of brisk walking on three days for each week you have to miss your tennis? If you meet that goal, give yourself a definite reward each day and at the end of each week.

Listed below are several points to consider in making your self-plan. The list is not exhaustive; you will have issues of your own to include, but it can give you a general framework to start work.

1. Generally stress seeking pleasures other than food. This principle seems especially important during the holiday seasons. Emphasize making the holiday special in ways that do not involve food. Whether you are religious or not, you can find ways to build your own or family traditions. This can focus on gifts, decorations, music, church or synogogue attendance, helping the needy, games and activities, and so on. Yes, it takes thought and work, but the effort will be rewarded both in a richer holiday and in better ability to handle eating problems. Be especially aware of this point in planning social activities. Look for ways to be active with people, rather than just being with them. In cold climates this is more difficult, but still possible. For example, if you are having a party and typically focus your attention on food, drink, and conversation, try everything from singing and dancing to party games in order to reduce the need to fill the time and yourself with food.

2. When you do eat, stress quality rather than quantity. See how many ways you can reduce the calories in your favorite foods. Take small portions of everything you like and concentrate on sensuous eating. Really enjoy the tastes, smells, and textures. This means doing everything you can to eat slowly and in as relaxed an atmosphere as you can create.

3. Be prepared to assert yourself, especially at parties. Hostesses are especially sensitive at this time of year to rejections of their

food. If you can alert the hostess (or host) in advance of the party, you can reassure her and get her on your side. Rehearse to yourself, or aloud with someone else, ways to phrase a rejection in a manner that will be light and still compliment the chef. But be prepared to be firm if he or she retaliates with further urging to indulge.

Another side of assertion is asking those around for what you want. A special family conference early in the season might be of great help. You can review the kinds of food to have, the help you need in preparing and cleaning up, and the kind of special reassurance you need to reinforce your efforts to control eating.

4. Here are a few more points about parties. Don't arrive overly hungry or thirsty. Have an advance idea of how much you would like to allow yourself to eat; some reduced intake in the day or days before can help, but don't starve yourself. Analyze how alcohol affects your eating. A bit may relax you and help you avoid nervous munching, but at some point alcohol will cloud your judgment and lead to overeating. Know your limits, and be prepared to search for drinks lower in calories (be sure you know how many calories are in eggnog, with and without alcohol!).

5. Beware of rush, tension, and fatigue. This season, especially with gift shopping and entertaining, often involves a great deal of extra work. Be sure to allow yourself time for complete relaxation. Know the early warning signals you experience when tension is building up and be prepared with noneating methods to relieve that tension.

6. If you are seeing family members or friends you do not see often, especially parents or grown-up children, take time in advance to review the kinds of conflicts you typically have with these people. What really ticks you off about their behavior? Then decide how you want to handle that behavior: Confront it and try to stop it, avoid it, or accept it (possibly smiling smugly to yourself). You may not be able to fully carry out this plan to cope with your mother-in-law's nagging or any other disturbance, but advance analysis and planning will improve your chances.

7. Anticipate the blues and the letdown. The folks don't call. The party is over. The gifts are all opened. When is it that you feel

low during this time of year? What can you do to give yourself pleasure at these times? Who can you talk to about the sadness?

8. Make New Year's resolutions, but don't be too hard on yourself. Everyone made mistakes; no one failed. Review your victories during the past weeks, and accept credit for them just as you accept responsibility for the mistakes. Minimize guilt; it will only make you feel bad and will get in the way of planning for the future. Make a new self-plan which will give you satisfactions in the coming weeks. If continued weight loss is your goal, make a plan that will be gradual even if you gained some weight during the holidays.

Some or all of these suggestions may be helpful to you, but the most important message is that the challenge of the holidays is complex and involves far more than your weight. Commit yourself to help yourself, but be easy—and above all, enjoy!

SUGGESTED PARTNER ACTIVITIES

The lesson this week introduces to your partner the idea that, at some point in time, she should be well enough in control of her eating to bring high-temptation foods back into her diet.

We have made the point to your partner that now may not be the time to reintroduce high-temptation foods. Whether or not your partner is ready to bring these foods back depends on her level of self-control skills. If she is habitually keeping accurate records of calories consumed and expended, has developed reliable stop-control skills, and in general has incorporated other skills to the point where they are routine, she has a good chance to master control of herself with those high-temptation foods.

If your partner is feeling strong enough to introduce these foods into her diet again, you can work on this with her. Important skills involve eating small amounts of the food, stopping and leaving some, and eating slowly, savoring the pleasure of eating such a pleasurable food. By eating some of the food with her this way yourself, you will be a model for your partner. More important, by joining her attempts to master high-temptation foods, you will be helping her change the guilt that many overweight people feel when they eat high-calorie foods in front of someone else. As long as the high-calorie food is eaten in a controlled manner (eaten in a planned portion that fits in with the daily calorie goal and recorded in the Food Diary), there is no reason to consider this mis-eating. Nevertheless, many overweight people feel that others seeing them eat the high-calorie food will believe they are cheating. Consequently, then tend to eat the high-calorie food in secret instead. Secret eating is usually dangerous. In addition, it is frequently followed by guilt. By staying by your partner's side if and when she decides to tackle these high-temptation foods, you will be participating in making secret eating less necessary for her.

chapter twelve
THE THREE-MARTINI LUNCH

Dark, cool, soft seats, a delightful escape from the office—an hour, or two if you're lucky, of wonderfully stimulating relaxation. Lunch—a time to mix business and pleasure; a time to hide, a time to be seen, to make contacts, to wrap up a deal. A tradition has grown up among businessmen and professionals that makes this meal a focal point of the entire day. There are the arrangements for people to share the meal, finding a place to go, making a reservation, even allowing a time to recover from the alcohol haze and overstuffed stupor that trail behind the magical meal.

Men use lunch to express all that is machismo in our middle-class world: holding our liquor, getting the right table from the maitre d', handling the waiter, controlling the conversation, seducing or selling table mates, and picking up the tab. The ritual is a new challenge each time, with alcohol and food to heighten the pleasure and take the edge off the anxiety that lurks behind every mis-spoken word, every lost deal, every embarrassing rejection. As women become more and more part of this world, the problems, as well as the glory, are shared. Social eating in restaurants presents a challenge for both sexes, whether the agenda includes business or not.

Whatever the benefits of lunch, with or without the three martinis, the problems raised and compounded by that tradition are tremendous. Aside from the calories (500–600 in the martinis alone), the food and drink cloud our minds for hours. Furthermore, we often arrive home to a laden table. Dinner is lunch all over again. By the time we get to our favorite chair in front of the TV we're lucky if we can stay awake long enough to have a bedtime snack.

"If I could just bring a brown bag lunch or eat at the little salad bar around the corner, I'd never have a weight problem." We hear this story and all of its sad variations over and over again in our weight-loss programs. It's very much related to the diet approach to weight control. If you could stick to a regimen, marching through life's many temptations with blinders on, you would have the willpower to keep from eating the wrong foods or just from eating too much. Many people get away with that for a while. They stay on the five-day wonder papaya and artichoke diet, and are overjoyed that they've lost ten pounds, or have even hung on until they reached their goal weight. Of course, how to arrange your life to keep it off is another story.

"What is willpower, anyway?" Willpower is eating lunch at the little salad bar around the corner. Or, is it eating only a salad at an important business lunch at Maxim's? Or, is it having only one martini or even only one potato chip?

We believe that it's all these things and more. It's not some mysterious force within you, somehow handed out, like blue eyes and blond hair, when the game begins. It's not even power in the sense of a unified strength that you gain by exercising. It's a collection of skills that everyone can learn and strengthen by practice. These skills are very much like a kit bag of tricks you can call on in time of need. Once you have decided to change something about yourself, you need all the tricks you can get. You have to practice them and be prepared to select the right ones for each challenging situation.

Now, let's return to lunch. You recognize that lunches in fancy restaurants are a problem for you. Being on a diet is one form of willpower, one trick in your bag. Similarly, avoiding business lunches is another possible technique. The difficulty with the avoidance technique is that it works too well. You knew you'd reach your goal if you could just stay away from trouble. It wasn't easy, but once done, it limited further temptations. If you could bring yourself to say to that prospect, "I'm sorry Jim, but we'll have to work out that deal at your office; I'm staying away from business lunches while I'm on my diet," you could eat your celery and artichokes in the peace and emptiness of your own office. But how long can you keep that up? And if you did keep it up until you reached goal weight, what now?

No, your will needs more than one power to win this war once and for all. You have to be able to go to a Maxim's for lunch, deal with the menu, the drinks, the gibes of your friends, the condescending waiter, the pastry cart rolling by—all of it. To do this means a careful analysis of yourself and the situation, some planning and some practice. It will be harder, at first, than relying only on the avoidance technique, but it is well worth the investment of effort.

THE GAME PLAN

Step One—Plan Ahead and Know the Territory

We've said that willpower is a collection of skills that you will be developing. Just as with any other skill, you can't expect to test yourself immediately under maximum challenge. It will take a little time before you're ready to handle with relative ease the most difficult restaurant situation.

Clearly the lunch problem is not all-or-none, eating carrots out of a brown bag in the office versus the most important deal of your life at the best restaurant in town. Try to make a list of several challenges, in order of difficulty. When you've worked on some willpower skills for these situations, you'll try them out in the easiest one first and work your way through the hierarchy. Table X shows a sample of how such a list might look.

Table X: List of Lunch Challenges in Order of Difficulty
1. Diet food alone at office.
2. Alone at a salad restaurant.
3. With a close friend (same sex) at a cafeteria.

4. With a friend (opposite sex) at an intimate café.
5. With a close associate at a fancy restaurant.
6. Important meal at a fancy restaurant with potential customer and his spouse.

You'll notice that such a list is highly individual and subjective. You might feel that item 3 would be more of a challenge for you than item 4. That's why each person has to devise his own list. There are many factors that go into making a situation easy or difficult—the restaurant, the sex of your dining partner(s), the availability of alcohol, and so on. The list could be lengthened considerably by adding more combinations of these factors. The important thing is that you have a sequence of steps that are in the right order for you. The idea is to try one step at a time. You will probably make errors. Going from step 3 to 4 may be a breeze, but you find step 5 too much to handle; maybe you'll have too much wine and say yes to the banana cream pie for dessert. Then you'll back up to step 4 again and do one or both of two things to succeed next time: Move step 5 higher on the list or add one or two intermediate steps between 4 and 5. For example, it might be wise to try that intimate café first with a same-sex friend who doesn't drink alcohol.

As you plan your list, select the territory very carefully. If you're not familiar with the restaurants you'll be using, take the time to stop by and just glance over the menus. Make sure you select locations where you have the kind of choices you'll feel most comfortable with. Life won't always allow you to stick to your gradual self-training plan, but with effort you can arrange things for a few weeks to try this step-by-step approach.

Step Two—Psych Out the Opposition

Below we list a series of subproblems in the restaurant-lunch challenge. Some or all of these may be important for you to solve; you may have others to add.

1. How hungry do I feel?
2. How much and what kind of food do I want to eat?
3. What does alcohol do to me?

4. How do the other people at the table affect my eating?
5. How does the waiter or waitress affect my eating?
6. Can I apply special eating techniques?
7. How do I feel afterward?

In Chapter 4 we saw how time is a major factor in solving most eating problems. The restaurant challenge is no exception. We tend to see a problem only in the immediate context. "I'm in Maxim's with the menu in front of me; what do I do now?" Your ability to control yourself in a particular restaurant is in part a function of what you did well in advance of stepping through the front door.

If you know that on a certain day you will be going out to lunch, some other advance work may help a great deal. Depending on weight fluctuations, you can save up calories for the occasion. For example, on a calorie-counting approach, you might decide to cut back two hundred calories a day for two or three days in advance, and plan to make up the rest of any deficit caused by the splurge by cutting back for several days after the luncheon and/or by some extra physical activity over that period. Most of the time you can make it clear to yourself that you won't be eating full dinners on days that you have a large lunch. Chapter 14 discusses working through these issues with your family.

On the day of the luncheon you might decide not to be saving calories. In fact, it might prove effective to eat more that morning than usual, so that you don't arrive at the restaurant feeling deprived and ravenous. You can also be careful not to be thirsty when you arrive. A tall glass of water or a cup of hot liquid in advance may reduce the amount of alcohol you consume.

Now you're ready to leave your office. Is there anything else you can do in advance? You can review the kinds of challenges you expect and have some strategies that you've planned in advance. Also, you can examine how you're feeling. If you're very tense and know that tension leads you to overeat, you can take a few minutes to slow down, unwind, and relax. The antistress strategies you learned in Chapter 7 will come in very handy at this time.

You've arrived at the restaurant (hopefully one you've selected, with a choice of foods appropriate to your diet). The other members of your party are also there. You first response, perhaps even at a bar before you're seated, may be vital to your sense of control throughout the meal—and it's that *sense* of control that you're aiming for, even more than a perfect victory over the food. Furthermore, a sense of control over the people may determine control of the food.

Time can be your ally. As much as possible, throughout the experience, arrange a relaxed pace. Give yourself time to psych out the other people you're with, time to consider the menu carefully, time to eat and drink slowly. Above all, allow time to be aware of what you're feeling and doing.

CHALLENGES IN THE GAME

Your first challenge at a restaurant is to be aware of your table partners—your relationship and attitudes toward them, their moods, the emotions they stimulate in you, their weights, their eating styles. Being aware will help you to maximize your sense of control.

GETTING THE UPPER HAND

Many people eat more when they're tense. Anything you can do to label your tension will enable you to try various coping techniques and reduce the need to use food as a tranquilizer. If, for example, you're with a person who is known for snobbish expertise about food and wine, your having selected a familiar restaurant enables you to feel comfortable with your knowledge of the menu and wine list. By communicating that familiarity at the outset, you may disarm any efforts by this person to put you down.

One of the most important issues in these first moments of contact is whether and when to mention that you're concerned with limiting yourself in some way. Some people never feel comfortable revealing this fact, especially in a situation where power is important. You too may take that position, and it's a legitimate one. However, at least consider the alternative strategy of using an announcement of your concern about diet as a ploy. This has the basic advantage of your having to make fewer excuses and refusals during the meal. But in addition, you will probably gain either sympathy or admiration, or both.

There was a time when eating and drinking great amounts was a symbol of wealth and power. Men were judged as big in both the literal and figurative sense. Perhaps as a carry-over from women who have valued being slim as an ideal for many generations, men have more recently moved toward the same standard. Restraint in eating and drinking is more often seen as a sign of a personal control, which is believed to generalize to other spheres, including business or professional skills.

It's important to present your position with confidence. Avoid expressing doubts, and never present your current effort as one in a long list of failed diets.

ALCOHOL STRATEGIES

Whether you've revealed your position early in the conversation or not, your first decision point is likely to be about drinks. It's important to understand the effects of alcohol and to plan a strategy for handling the stuff.

Alcohol is a mind-altering drug. If it came in tablets or had to be injected, Prohibition would probably never have been repealed. The fact that it is consumed in a tasty liquid form is essential for its popularity and acceptability. Unfortunately, this form makes it a double problem for the weight-conscious person: 1) Alcohol and its mixers contain calories, and 2) drinking it clouds your judgment about overeating.

As a drug, alcohol is a depressant. This might come as a surprise to you. Many of us drink to get rid of depression, to loosen our inhibitions. By depressing the top part of the brain first, we get this paradoxical antidepressant effect because our depressed cortex allows us to forget and to stop worrying.

Unfortunately, not worrying includes not worrying about what we eat or drink. So we lose track of the peanuts, chips, dip, etc., and we lose track of the number of drinks we have consumed.

This problem is made worse by the way we consume alcohol. Especially in bars or restaurants, we often cannot be sure of the amount of alcohol in mixed drinks. To make matters worse, variations in our stomach contents will affect our reaction to the alcohol. All of this makes for a situation difficult to control.

Despite this gloomy picture, you may still want to drink. For some people the drug has some benefits which offset the problems. For one thing, if you eat more when you're tense, the relaxing effect of alcohol could actually help you to eat less. So, short of total abstention, you can try some of these techniques to limit yourself:

1. Maximize your control over portions by selecting drinks with known quantities (e.g., wine, beer, straight hard liquor). Avoid elaborate, and often high-calorie, concoctions.

2. Even within standard drinks, there are calorie choices. White wine has fewer calories than sweet reds. Low-calorie beers are now widely available.

Table of Alcoholic Drink Calorie Values*

Beer	12 oz. container	150
Light beer	12 oz. container	100
Cocktails	3 oz. glass	200
Highball	8 oz. glass	250
Wine		
dry	4 oz. glass	100
sweet	4 oz. glass	150

*These are average values, rounded off for easy use.

3. If having something to drink in your hand at all times is important, like at a cocktail party, try alternating alcoholic and nonalcoholic rounds.

4. Chapter 5 shows you how to eat more slowly as a technique to improve your ability to judge hunger and satisfaction. The same principle applies to alcohol. Don't drink because you're thirsty; use other low-calorie beverages for that. Drink alcohol slowly and train yourself to be aware of the psychological state you're in. Notice how you get fuzzy after so many ounces of a given form of alcohol. Can you tell from speech, the way you laugh, your skin tempera-

ture, your vision? Remember, alcohol is a drug. You be the doctor, and set your safe dosage. Confidence in your ability to control will enable you to relax and enjoy the amount you choose. This certainly seems a worthwhile goal in the context of that important luncheon.

"ARE YOU READY TO ORDER, SIR?"

Recently, we went to a restaurant with a weight-conscious friend. After staring at the menu for a while, she said, "How much does a corned beef sandwich cost?" I looked up, puzzled, and said, "Isn't the price printed on your menu?" She laughed and explained what she meant: "How many calories will it cost me?" Whether you're actually on a calorie-counting program or not, it would be useful to have the numbers as a relative guide to help you make choices. You then can literally ask yourself, "How much can I afford today?" Or, "Am I willing to save two hundred calories by having tomato juice as an appetizer instead of creamy clam chowder, and then use the two hundred later toward a dessert?" While you may want to appear generous with your money, you can be a veritable tightwad with calories. "Baked potato; no butter and no sour cream. Steak, but just four ounces please, and no butter or sauce on it. Leave the avocado off the special salad."

THE INTIMIDATING WAITER

There's a rule to restaurant life: The higher the prices, the more arrogant the waiters. You would think that a larger chunk out of your wallet, especially for the tip, would entitle you automatically to better service. On the contrary, waiters in fancy restaurants often seem to identify with the owners and the chefs, and are seldom anxious to cater to the dietary whims of us poor slobs paying the bills. So you've got to demand your rights, politely (at least at first) but firmly. The list of graduated situations that you develop may help you here. As you increase the difficulty of your restaurant encounters from the point of view of the company and type of restaurant, also gradually escalate your willingness to make special requests of the waiters.

The ultimate sense of power comes from sending something back to the kitchen if it doesn't meet your order. Some people are so cowed by waiters that they have never done this and would rather eat and pay for food that is completely unsatisfactory. This form of assertiveness is so important that if you are unable to do it, we urge you to rehearse at home and even get a friend to role play a waiter for you. In addition to the relevance for calories consumed, assertiveness with the waiter will make you feel better about yourself, more relaxed and confident, and hence less in need of food as a tranquilizer. Chapter 15 goes into greater detail on techniques for increasing assertiveness.

A final few words about ordering the food. Don't feel bound by the menu. If there is a food you want that doesn't appear, ask for it. After years of passively accepting hash brown potatoes with our breakfast eggs, we noticed someone asking to substitute sliced tomatoes. The waitress gave him a dirty look, but he got what he wanted. And now so do we! Also, feel free to order à la carte and to order from any part of the menu at any time. We have been to elegant restaurants where we had a whole meal of appetizers. Once we ordered a hot appetizer and said we would decide on the rest of the meal later. After the appetizer, we ordered dessert. In many restaurants these tactics will not win smiles from the waiter. But if you cultivate your favorite restaurant, there will be no problem. Anyway, the other people at your table will probably order more "normally" and get you off the hook. As an added bonus, you'll gain a conversation edge and the admiration of your table mates.

EAT SENSUOUSLY AND
LEAVE A LITTLE
FOR THE CHILDREN STARVING IN INDIA

All of the suggestions we make to you in other chapters about eating slowly and sensuously apply with special force in restaurants. The distraction of the restaurant and the conversation will take your attention away from your body. You may find that the first bite of some dish tastes fantastic, especially if you've been kept waiting too long. Then you get to talking and you're suddenly on automatic pilot, filling the fork well before the mouth is empty, keeping up a steady stream of food and drink. Unless you make a conscious effort to attend to the food and its effect on you, you will lose control.

There are a number of techniques useful in this effort. If you tend to be a fast eater, notice the eating rates of those around you. Choose the slowest eater and pace yourself to her. (It's usually a woman; they tend to eat more daintily.) If necessary, put your utensils down every few bites and wait a few seconds before you begin again.

Talk about the food. You may want to get on with business, if that's the purpose of the meal, but try to resist being impetuous. Often, you will gain by delay. The old aristocratic custom we see in movies was to postpone business until brandy and cigars, often in another room. Perhaps we can't go that far, but it's worth an effort to enjoy the food first.

We have recommended that you learn to leave food on your plate. Although restaurants often serve oversized portions, the pressure to clean your plate seems even greater than at home. First of all, there's the cost. Many people live out the delusion that they can only get their money's worth if they eat it all. The restaurant never gets the message that the portions are too large, and continues to pile it on the plates and on the bill. Then there's the authority vested in the waiter, who comes to represent our parents, silently admonishing us to save the starving millions by eating more. Sometimes he does so not so silently. We've had a waiter literally trail us to the door of the restaurant demanding to know why we were leaving the cheesecake. There really is a great sense of satisfaction when you see the look of wonderment on the faces of everyone within earshot of your reply, "It's excellent, but I've just had enough."

There is the twenty-minute-lag rule we explained in Chapter 5. If you eat until you are satisfied, you will feel full in about twenty minutes. If you eat until you are full, you'll feel uncomfortably stuffed in twenty minutes.

GETTING A HANDLE ON CAFETERIAS
AND SMORGASBORDS

Before we leave restaurants, a few words about cafeterias and smorgasbords. These places have two advantages. First, you have much more control over what you take; and second, you can break up the meal with walks back to the line. Ideally, the more decision points, the better able you are to control yourself. However, there are obvious pitfalls. A cafeteria, by its structure, urges you to buy all of your food at once. Deserts are put first in the line, to assure that you'll buy.

The smorgasbord feeds on your greed. If your mother ever told you, "Your eyes are bigger than your stomach," here's the place to prove she was wrong. The skill with which some people pile their plates and get safely back to their table would be the envy of many a circus performer. The answer to the problem requires a relatively simple mental switch, from quantity to variety. If you can view the smorgasbord as a challenge to see how many distinctive tastes you can experience, the quantity challenge disappears. Go back as many times as you want, so long as the foods are in very small quantities. Aim to see plate on all sides of each little pile of food.

chapter thirteen
THE POWER
OF POSITIVE BINGEING

"Why did I do it—why, oh why did I suddenly lose control and eat every tempting food I could lay my hands on?"

Let's start by looking at the answers to this question in this chapter on The Binge. The first and most important thing every person prone to bouts of binge eating should realize is that there *are* answers.

The binge doesn't "just happen." It happens for a specific or, more frequently, for a variety of reasons.

Once you begin to look at your binge eating, you will be able to see clearly exactly when and why you are likely to begin an eating binge. We have already discussed conditions that affect start controls and stopping controls. The situations and principles are similar for controlling a binge. There are two categories to consider: first, your environment, and second, your own feelings or mood.

In the first category, think about environmental circumstances or common situations that could start off a binge for you. For example, some people tend to feel prone to binge on a particular day, like blue Mondays, or when they are bored or alone. Or maybe gray weather will do it for you. Some women have a regular binge just before a menstrual period.

Now, add the second category. People with a weight problem are inclined to binge—probably more frequently than for any other reason—when they are feeling in some way rejected, when some human relationship has taken a downturn or simply when they are not in close human contact with another person.

A classic situation was reported by a client a short time ago. The woman had recently been divorced and had not yet formed any new steady relationship with a man. She described one particular time when she and a woman friend went out on a Saturday evening to a dance. The evening was not a social disaster; she was asked to dance a number of times. Nevertheless, the two of them left feeling somewhat discouraged and lonely.

Back at home, when her friend had departed, she began to feel what she described as "terribly bad." What she did was to begin to eat—and continue to eat and eat throughout the next few days.

Now the explanation was that she simply wasn't getting what she wanted. Her body was acutely sensitive to this and reacted to it.

However your own life situation may be different, there are bound to be times and situations when your needs are not fully satisfied. There are going to be drizzly days, boring or lonely days. These conditions may combine with a particular personal problem to create an explosive mixture.

THE VITAL EARLY WARNING SIGNALS

The key to success in controlling binge eating is to have some preventative strategies and to get the upper hand by starting these strategies early, thereby getting time on your side.

At the moment you begin a binge, your spirits and self-control are at their lowest ebb. Besides the feeling of frustration or depression, you probably have a certain apathy about it all. Even if a friend suggested something more beneficial, like going for a walk, chances are your answer would be "No way!" It may be too late to do something constructive at this point. You're already on your way.

So, instead of letting things go to this advanced stage, it is important to pay attention to all the early warning signals that begin to build up into a binge.

Sometimes, as soon as you wake up in the morning, you are aware of an early warning signal that might say that you slept badly, or that your stomach is upset, or there's a hectic, tightly scheduled day ahead. While binges are more likely to start at night, the signs signaling their possible approach can usually be detected early in the morning or at the moment when a day that may have started off well suddenly takes its first downturn.

These signals that you are in for a miserable evening ahead are a call for immediate action. Don't sink into inertia and apathy. It will be difficult to do something positive—but positive action is just as essential as your diet. What can you do, specifically?

Here are some strategies to beat the pre-binge mood.

You need a battle plan, a series of preventative actions you can use when binge signals are detected on the horizon. Write out your personal plan, and put it up in a place where you are likely to see it and use it when the crisis begins.

STRATEGY 1.   Plan something enjoyable.

We have found that at this pre-binge stage many people are amazingly blocked in their ability to initiate things that can give them pleasure and enjoyment. The techniques discussed in Chapter 9 for increasing the range and availability of pleasures may prove especially vital in heading off a binge.

STRATEGY 2.   Physical exercise combats depression.

In Chapter 6 we explained the remarkable mood-lifting effect of physical exercise. If you can persuade yourself to walk or run or exercise, it is quite likely that this alone will combat your binge mood; it will do wonders for your state of mind. Observe yourself and you will see that the more depressed you get, the slower you get, until you stop moving altogether. Get your body moving!

STRATEGY 3.   Do something virtuous.

If you have a hard time thinking of pleasures for yourself, try to think of something useful to do instead of succumbing to a binge-prone evening. If you are convinced that you are in for an unpleasant time, you might as well attack some of those nasty jobs that have been nagging at you. The aftermath could be a warm glow of achievement that could shift your mood. Just be sure that your virtuous feelings don't turn toward food as a reward!

STRATEGY 4.   Attend to your emotions.

Refer to Chapter 8 for a detailed discussion of emotions. To review briefly here, when you detect warning signals of a binge, take time to reflect on what unexpressed emotions you may be confusing with hunger. Consider whether direct expression of emotions toward the person(s) stimulating some private release of emotional tension would be more appropriate for you right now. Finally, see if talking to someone about your feelings will relieve some of the tension.

WHEN ALL ELSE FAILS: EAT!

Each of you has your own special definition of a binge. For some it is eating three cookies in midafternoon. For others it means drawing the drapes, withdrawing to bed, and eating for three days until no more food is left in the house. Regardless of what magnitude of mis-eating your particular definition involves, the phenomenon of binge eating can be examined and controlled, using the same techniques we have been practicing up until now.

Although we all would like to be assured that having better tools and knowledge will *always* give us the upper hand and prevent mis-eating, it is important to be realistic and know that there will be occasions when temptation looms too large. On those occasions, when everything goes wrong, you just feel like following Oscar Wilde's advice when he said, "The only way to deal with temptation is to give in."

We will now discuss strategies that will allow you to *safely* give in to temptation when all else has failed. We will teach you how to convert a binge from a totally uncontrolled experience to one that we will call constructive mis-eating.

Let's look at the *before, during,* and *after* of binging. How can the eating experience be limited and controlled?

BEFORE

"What Do I Really Want to Eat Right Now?"

If you've tried or ruled out other strategies to avoid mis-eating and have decided that eating is unavoidable, you owe it to yourself to eat the right thing. You see, cravings don't happen by accident. Often we have learned to associate particular foods with relief from discomfort or with the feeling of pleasure. This association may go back to early childhood experiences. We've all heard jokes and stories about the mother who feeds her children a particular ethnic dish whenever they're not feeling well (chicken soup cures anything). We have special foods to keep out the cold (porridge?), special foods to keep cool. Special foods are healthy, make us strong. Then there are all of the foods associated with joyous occasions (breads, cakes, sweets). Or maybe you had your own specialty for a lonely rainy afternoon (peanut butter sandwiches?).

When you have decided you are going to mis-eat, how can you pick the right food? Try this sequence: Sit down, relax (as we've taught you), and let your mind wander. As your imagination works, foods will pop into your head. Focus on a food as it occurs to you; imagine it as vividly as you can; even imagine eating it, how it will taste. As you do this, you'll find yourself rejecting some foods outright, considering a few, and finally one will seem just right.

If you're having trouble, remind yourself of your mood. By then you should have gone through the process of analyzing what's bothering you and labeling any emotions you might be experiencing. Sometimes we find that certain foods go with specific emotions and can help to relieve the tensions of these emotions. For example, suppose you're angry. Possibly the best kind of food for you would be something chewy or crunchy— something you could "really get your teeth into," to relieve the angry tension in your mouth and jaw. Maybe you're lonely, really feeling empty. Then something warm and filling, like a hearty soup, might be best. (If this is beginning to sound like a television commercial, it's no accident; the advertising copywriters have made an art of appealing to these special needs in people.)

You might want to prepare for such occasions now by making

a list of your favorite foods. Next to each, write down what situations or emotions they might work best for. Try to remember times in the past when these foods helped you. As you prepare the list, be aware of exactly what characteristics of the food you really like. Is it the crust of the rye bread or the soft center? Is it the crunchiness of the nuts or the saltiness? Milk chocolate or bittersweet? The hamburger or the bun? This will help you to get *exactly* what you want when you decide to go after it. Also, you may be able to minimize calories a bit by being very specific (for example, by eating bread crusts and not the centers).

Plan

A binge is upon you (preventative action has failed). You've decided on what will be best to eat, and you're now ready to plan your binge. You may have to shop for the exact food you want, but it's worth the effort. If what you want is best gotten at a restaurant, and you can manage that, then arrange to go out to eat (be aware of the restaurant problems discussed in Chapter 12). Try to get a friend or relative to share this experience with you. You may or may not want to reveal how you're feeling, but you know it will help *not to mis-eat alone*.

If you're eating at home, it's not enough just to get the right food; you have to prepare it really well and create the right mood for enjoying it—a beautiful table setting, even candles and flowers. Treat this as a special occasion; really spoil yourself. Make sure as many distractions as possible are avoided.

DURING

Enjoy

This is a time when your slow-eating exercises will really help. Enjoy every morsel of this special food. Eat it slowly, sensuously, experiencing all the sensation you can from each mouthful. Make this a total eating experience.

For example, instead of eating the ice cream from the carton, take a small portion, put it in a bowl, and decorate it with your favorite toppings. Put the rest away and bring your portion to the table. Sit down and enjoy it. Close your eyes and taste every spoonful to the fullest.

Whether your chosen food is ice cream, something crunchy, or something spicy, the important thing is to get the most pleasure possible from the eating of it. *Enjoy it!*

AFTER

Minimize Guilt

Let's start with a simple rule: Guilt is bad. If most overweight people know that they eat when they feel bad, then they know that they eat even more when they feel guilty. One of the most important factors in *lengthening* a binge is feeling guilty and saying to yourself something like, "I've blown it; I might as well keep on eating." How can you stop feeling guilty when you've been conditioned to believe that overeating is piggish, weak-willed, bad? The key to changing this attitude is the phrase, "Self-control means I always have another choice." Each moment—between bites, between servings, between boxes, between trips out to the store, between orders in the restaurant—provides you with a choice, a chance to stop eating and begin anew. Freedom means having a lot of choices, but it also means taking the responsibility to make your choices.

The moment when you break a chain of strong, almost automatic responses during a binge, when you switch from being passive to taking an active role again in your life, is a moment of great victory. *It's a moment of pride and no time to feel guilty.* You've turned the tide—and the further it has crept up on you, the greater the achievement.

If guilt feelings are persistent, try boosting your positive feelings about yourself. Sit down with pencil and paper and list ways in which you have changed, things you can do now that you couldn't before, victories you have had.

Instead of hitting yourself on the head or labeling yourself a failure, try saying "I'm only human, and sometimes the going is just too rough."

Recognize the difference between name-calling or labeling and constructive self-criticism. Experts on child rearing point out the importance of how a parent reacts to misbehavior. A parent who gets angry and says how he feels about *specific* behavior ("I don't like your doing that") is constructive. Using labels ("You're a brat," "You're no good," etc.) is destructive. It lowers the child's self-esteem and prevents his taking the right steps to change his behavior. The same principle seems to apply when we deal with ourselves. After all, part of all of us is still that little child, wanting its way, rebellious. The "parent" part of us wants to punish, criticize, make the "child" feel guilty. In between is the real adult who can be rational and compromise and say, in effect, "Okay, you've made a mistake; now what are you going to do about it?"

Notice this distinction in the way you react to other people (adults and children) and to yourself during the coming week. See if you can minimize labeling and generalizing. Try to react only to the behavior that's occurring right at the moment.

Replan

Once you've stopped the mis-eating situation, counted the damage, and dealt with your guilt, the last stage is the most important. Review the binge—what led up to it, what were the early signals, what choices did you have to deal with it at various times along the way, what strategies did you try, how did they work, where did they go wrong, when will similar situations be likely to occur again? Plan new strategies for next time. Search for ways to shorten the mis-eating, so that you have one half of a binge or one quarter of a binge next time. You can outline your analysis and post it somewhere to help you when the next signals occur, to be aware of all the alternatives available to you.

You should try to record all you've eaten on your Food Diary and attempt to compensate. However, don't use your calorie count as a form of penance. You can only make up a reasonable number of calories in the next few days. It would be a mistake to starve yourself or go on an especially stringent regime. Your goal should be to get back to normal, controlled eating as soon as possible, but not to overreact and make reestablishing control too discouraging.

SUMMARY ON BINGES

When tensions build up and can't be handled and mis-eating of larger proportions threatens, we call it a binge. The strategy we've been describing advises you to resist as far as you are able, and then—if you can't prevent it—to give in, but to give in in a very special, *very controlled* way—a way that will perhaps limit the quantity and duration of the binge. Your goal in regard to this kind of serious mis-eating should be twofold: 1) Picking up the signals of prebinge tension as early as possible to take prevention action, and 2) limiting the binge as much as possible.

chapter fourteen
A LITTLE HELP
AROUND THE HOUSE

There are many different life-styles led by the people reading this book. Some of you live alone, some with friends, some with families. Various parts of what follows will be relevant to many of you; make use of what would be most helpful. Even if you live alone, you relate to friends in connection with eating and can profit from many of the points discussed.

The following is a kind of problem checklist. Read through it first and check off which items are most relevant to you, then review each checked item carefully to decide what you need to do about that point.

1. *Whom to tell.* You've dieted many times and suffered from the comments of friends and family: "What, again?" "Another diet?" "You'll never be thin!" "Give it up," "Why don't you just use a little willpower?" You may be tempted to hide this new effort and see if you can do it alone, then surprise them all. We feel strongly that your weight and what you eat are your own business and your own responsibility. No one should be losing weight under pressure from anyone else. However, now that you have decided to lose weight and to learn the skills presented in this book, you can seek out the kind of help from friends and family that you need and want. Telling the people you feel are important and can be

helpful is often a boost to your motivation. This is especially true for the people living in your household. When you have read through the following points and checked those needing work, we suggest you have a *family conference*. At a time convenient to everyone concerned, meet to tell them what you are doing and how you want them to help you. Get their commitment to work with you and iron out any misunderstandings related to food, meals, or any of the other points discussed below.

2. *The shape of those around you.* Let's first look at the case of the spouse or other close adult living with you who is noticeably thin. It would be only natural for you to feel a certain amount of envy, even resentment, toward this person. He or she might be a "natural thinny," one of those lucky people who never seems to bother about his weight, eating whatever and whenever he pleases. These people, we find, are relatively rare, especially over the age of thirty. There are other types of thin people, though: the person who eats a regular and fairly limited diet, or the one who eats heavily in spurts and then diets down a few pounds, or the one who exercises heavily to offset heavy eating. It's important that you understand just how your friend or relative does it; ask him, if you're not sure, and discuss it with him. It's easy to assume that "it's just the way he is naturally," rather than looking for the causes just as you would look for the causes of your being over-weight. This person can be an important source of information for you, both by talking to you and by your observing him, or even by joining or imitating him. For example, you may find that your thin friend or spouse is a much slower eater than you. Notice *how* he slows down. Does he toy with his food? Does he take small bites? Does he drink a lot of liquid between bites? Observe these small details and try adjusting to his pace. Maybe your spouse is more active and takes a walk after dinner in the evening—this is a golden opportunity for togetherness and an increase in your energy output if you can join him. Maybe your roommate sleeps fewer hours than you, rising an hour earlier to get household chores done before going to work. Don't assume you need as much sleep as you're getting until you try slightly less and see how it feels. Always be open to experimenting with your lifestyle.

Let's now take a look at the opposite problem, a relative or friend at home who is also noticeably overweight. A critical issue here is whether he or she is involved in trying to reduce or is apparently satisfied with his or her present weight. If he is not trying to reduce and you want him to, try getting this issue openly discussed and resolved, saying exactly what you would like from him or her. If he is trying to reduce, then cooperation is the key, and you should be working together on food plans, eating patterns, and any other topic that could be mutually helpful. You might have thought of a competition in weight loss. We shy away from that strategy, especially between husbands and wives. Men seem to have a slight physical advantage in weight-loss efforts. In any case, the advantage to the winner in any competition is probably more than offset by the frustration and disappointment for the loser. Stick to cooperative efforts; perhaps set a family reward for both partners reaching some goal along their own weight-reduction path.

3. *Physical surroundings.* In Chapter 4 we suggested that high-calorie foods be isolated in a separate cupboard or shelf, and labeled. You should discuss with the other members of your household the presence of these foods at this time. You may have the final goal of being able to eat controlled amounts of any foods, yet decide that you are not quite ready to be tempted by sweets or certain other high-calorie foods around the house. Say openly that you want a temporary withdrawal of these foods until you can work them safely back into your eating plans. It may be a difficult job to put yourself first and be assertive enough to say to your spouse and children, "I want you to help me by not bringing doughnuts or candy (or whatever the problem food is) into the house until I tell you I'm ready." But if they know you're sincerely seeking their help, most families will cooperate. If other members are also overweight, this strategy will help them, too.

4. *Sabotage.* Some friends or relatives will occasionally, consciously or unconsciously, try to sabotage your efforts—for example, by bringing a high-calorie sweet home. In one case a client told us that her husband told all of her friends, "Feed my wife, she's getting too thin." It may be that the spouse, or even roommate, is threatened in some way by your becoming slimmer and physically more attractive. An overweight spouse is, in a way, security against competition. You may feel comfortable discussing this

openly. Or you may want to take the less-direct approach of frequently reassuring your mate of your continuing affection for him or her. Specific acts of sabotage have to be firmly stopped, however. Again, a difficult act of assertiveness is called for: "Don't bring that kind of food for me right now. I know you're trying to do something nice, but gifts of food are too tempting for me."

5. *Nagging and producing guilt.* All of us resent being treated like children, especially since we all are still partly children and are likely to rebel against people who act like parents. A spouse or friend who nags may have all the good intentions in the world, but may do you great harm by making you feel rebellious or guilty, thereby leading you to eat even more. Often this parentlike behavior leads you to eat secretly, hiding from yourself and others. You must feel free to make your mistakes and be responsible for them. No matter how many times you have failed before, your spouse or friend can't take responsibility for you; it will do no good and may do harm. Discuss this openly and request at least a truce period of several months, during which he or she tries to take the pressure off you. Not nagging may be as big a feat of self-control for him as reduced eating is for you. So bear with his gritted teeth and frowns as he tries not to nag. The next section will help by giving you some ideas of positive ways that he can now help you.

A word about real parents, especially if they live with you (or you with them). These may be the people who started you on your way to being overweight. You may resent this, and they may feel guilty about it. As hard as it may be, you must try to treat that as history and work toward an adult relationship with your parents. Getting an overzealous mother to stop pushing food (especially food she cooked) on her now grown-up son or daughter is no easy trick. We've even had clients who had to say, "Mom, until I get my weight under control, I've got to stay away from your good cooking; it's just too tempting." Usually, gentle but firm resistance will work with a parent who is probably genuinely concerned that you lose weight. Occasionally, a parent or spouse feels you shouldn't lose weight, that fat is healthy—a tougher situation! Again, your conference task is to firmly state your own goals and to make clear that you are an adult and are going to choose your own weight and eating patterns.

6. *Ways to get help and support.* As important as stopping negative

behavior is starting to get some positive responses from spouse, family, and friends. Examine your own desires carefully and present them clearly in the family conference. Here are a few ideas for your consideration.

a. *Focus on the positive*. We've discussed above the importance of minimizing nagging and criticism. The relative or friend who wants to help may need to be told when to praise, even how to praise. As you go through this book, you will be practicing many new techniques of self-control. Some of these will be visible and can be praised; for example, eating more slowly, leaving food on your plate, refusing a snack, taking a walk, learning calorie values, and so on. The friend or relative should be totally unconcerned with *what* you eat (unless you *ask* him or her to help, for example, with learning calories) but can praise you for positive changes in all of these other areas. You can even tell him what to say ("Wow, you're terrific!"), or better yet, to give you a big hug whenever you suggest you go out for a walk after dinner. You can plan specific rewards together for making progress toward your goal—a movie, shopping, even dinner out.

If you've struggled with your weight for years, you know that it's mostly a lonely problem. But you can ask for help and support from those around you who care. We have given you a number of specific ways to get that help. The first time it may be hard to ask, but it will be worth the effort.

b. *Physical activities are more fun with company*. If you can find a form of recreation to do together, even walking, it will be more fun and more likely that you will do it regularly.

c. *A discreet word about sex*. This is a tough area to discuss openly. We don't believe that overweight people have any more or fewer sexual problems than anyone else. If you do, and feel that counseling will help, seek it out. You may have a simple communication problem about what you want and when. Again, this is difficult for many of us to talk about, but the pain of the first discussion may be worth it in avoiding sexual frustrations that are leading you to mis-eat.

d. *Practical help around the house.* You can get help with meal planning, shopping, cooking, and cleaning up. This may be for the general purpose of relieving strain for you, or may help you specifically with difficult times. For example, if you are prone to eat leftovers from plates as you do the dishes, having your spouse working alongside you will reduce considerably the likelihood of this behavior. We have urged you to find a regular time each day to relax. It's up to you to get the cooperation of your household to get that time and that privacy you will need. This is especially important for the person who works outside the home, but also for those of you who work at home; it can be even more important for those with children (who can be given more responsibility to help out). One of our clients described how she came from work at five, was rushed by the children immediately with all their demands and all their problems, felt compelled to get right down to work preparing an evening meal, felt tired and tense, and nibbled for a solid hour as she worked in the kitchen. We urged her to make clear to her family that her new, *real* arrival time was five-thirty. The lady who came in the door at five was not to be disturbed for at least a half hour while she took a shower, a nap, read the newspaper, or did whatever she needed to do to relax. This half hour paid off a double dividend: She no longer felt the need to nibble, and she had much more energy to enjoy her family for the rest of the evening.

e. *Being sensitive to your feelings.* Someone living with you often knows when you are depressed or tense, but may feel helpless about it. Discuss what he or she might do. Often the simple question, "Would you like to talk?" or "Can I do anything to help?" or "You seem sad (or tense)" is enough to allow you to express what's bothering you and discuss what can be done about it. If you're like many of us, your first reaction is to wall yourself off and say, in one way or another, "Just leave me alone." You can discuss with your family the possibility that it's okay for them to persist and try to draw you out when this happens. Just letting you know they care enough to persist may bring you out of your shell.

f. *Physical and social activity.* One sure way to get you out of feeling *down* is for a relative or friend to get you active. Discuss new activities to do together, especially physical things (dancing is great). Doing these regularly is important, but also you can use them as techniques to raise your spirits at bad times.

g. *Helping someone else helps you.* One good topic for a household conference is ways for reciprocal helping. Your friend or relative may not have a weight problem, but may have other problems you can help with. Trade off. You will get great satisfaction helping him or her, and at the same time will improve your communication about the helping process.

7. *Helping your children to stay slim or get slim.* Many overweight adults are aware of the ways their own parents contributed to their weight problem and are working hard to prevent the problem from being carried on to the next generation. Still, some of you feel compelled to overfeed your growing child and to provide him with high-calorie foods that will make him so unhappy to be without. While young children probably don't need diets (your doctor should advise you about this), they also don't need an excess of sweets, fats, and fried foods. Discuss this openly in the conference. In addition to temporary restrictions to help you, your whole household should consider changes in eating style that would promote health for everyone. There are some principles gleaned from our research and observation of overweight people that may help you to prevent obesity in your children. The principles are not necessarily easily carried out, but you can take the first step of considering them and giving them a try.

a. *Forget "Clean your plates"*—While you want to encourage children to try new foods and a wide variety of foods, in the end it will be attractive preparation that will encourage them to eat well. Cleaning up your plate is not good economics if doing so leads you to overeat and acquire a larger and larger appetite as you grow older. You would do better to return to an older philosophy of "It's good manners to leave a little on your plate." Children can show they appreciated the cooking by *saying so*, not by eating too much of it.

b. *Don't ever encourage a child to eat if he says he's not hungry.* You might have a rule about not eating sweets after he says he's not hungry for dinner. But always encourage a child to be sensitive to his hunger and satisfaction signals so that he carries this sensitivity into adulthood. It's even okay to skip meals. Children have a way of balancing their own diets, if given the chance. Of course, you must set your own limits about preparing food for a child at all odd hours, but it's usually possible to arrange an easy, healthful snack later for a child who wants to skip a meal.

c. *Don't rush a child's eating.* Let him play with his food; that may be messy, but enjoyable. Slow, *enjoyable* eating is much better than fast, tense eating in preventing a pattern of compulsiveness that leads to obesity later in life.

d. *Do not reward with food or punish by depriving food.* Look for other rewards and punishments. As much as possible, avoid giving food this extra meaning. Whatever good foods you serve should not be seen as linked to being a good or bad child. This seems to lead to an undue importance being attached to food when we reach adulthood, especially to sweets.

e. *Encourage every form of physical activity that your child seems to enjoy.* If your child seems sluggish or lacking in interest in physical activity, ask your doctor about it and look for new activities that will interest the child. As you know, lack of physical activity is as much a cause of obesity as overeating.

WORKING WITH A PARTNER

At the end of Chapter 3 we suggested that a more formalized system of partner participation may be useful to you in your weight-loss efforts. As a beginning of such a partnership we suggest you have your prospective partner (he/she need not be a spouse) read the following letter and then discuss the points in this chapter of most concern to you. From there, if he or she is willing, we urge reading the chapters as you go along and trying some of the specific suggestions for partner participation at the end of many of the chapters.

A LETTER TO YOUR PARTNER

(Originally published in *Slimming* magazine, Great Britain)

Dear Sir,

I can well appreciate that you have reached the point where you now feel thoroughly bored and fed up with the whole subject of your wife's weight problem. I imagine that you have passed through the stages where you expressed your concern about her weight, urged her to slim and possibly acted as a kind of policeman who tried to guard her from the temptations of overeating. And all to no avail.

Having failed abysmally (or decided that she will fail abysmally whatever you do) you are now "turned off" to the whole problem. You may be surprised to hear this, but I think it is just as well that those stages of "trying to be helpful" have gone by. Often in a sincere effort to be helpful the husband gets over-involved and his well-intentioned criticism actually hinders his wife's efforts. This applies in very much the same way to a wife trying to get her husband to slim or a mother trying to get her daughter to slim—in fact, to any two people in a close family relationship.

My advice to anyone trying to act as a "slimming policeman" to any member of the family is first of all to back off, so that you can begin again from a more neutral position.

Criticism, even if well-intended, accurate and mildly stated, often has a most disastrous effect on the slimmer. While it may be accepted in a positive way from an outsider, like a doctor or slimming club leader, it rarely does anything but harm in a close family relationship.

By being critical because your wife has overeaten, you seem to set off a cycle of guilt, childlike rebellion, and renewed overeating. Your wife herself probably doesn't

156

realize why she reacts in this way. But it is largely due to the fact that we all bring into our adult makeup a certain amount of our childlike attitude—particularly our attitude towards parental authority.

From early childhood most of us have learned to associate eating with some conflict with our parents—whether about not eating enough, eating the wrong things, or eating too much. When a husband steps into this parental role he inadvertently encourages his wife to revert to a childlike role. And all children have an urge to rebel!

Often the adult person reacts just like many children caught in the act of misbehaving; she continues that act in secret. Most overweight people will admit (although only to themselves) that nearly all their excess eating is done not in public but when they are quite alone.

By being critical you are doing something even more dangerous than stimulating a subconscious sense of rebellion. You are increasing your wife's feeling of guilt. Whatever her outward attitude is, you can be certain that she will view overeating as a bad thing to do and feel guilty when she does it. Unfortunately the guilt, while it may temporarily suppress eating, seems very soon to increase overeating. Most women are most tempted to eat when they feel bad. Anyone feeling guilty is feeling bad. It's as simple as that. This paradox is a thorn in the side of many overweight wives. This is why you can never succeed as a watchdog "parent." But you can help as a fellow adult, reinforcing your wife's adult attitude to self-control.

Once you have accepted that you must stop being the critical "parent" and that the problem is basically your wife's responsibility, you will begin to reduce her feelings of guilt and rebelliousness towards you.

The next move is your wife's. Help which is requested is best received. When she feels confident that you will not be critical of her, she can then perhaps say: "I need your help." At that point, you can sit as two adults and discuss what kind of help she wants and how she feels that you can best respond to her problems.

While I cannot possibly design a plan for each couple—this must be individually worked out—I can describe some of the approaches that can be used successfully.

The first principle which seems important for all couples to establish is the substitution of praise for criticism.

Praise can be a powerful tool in helping a person to change, but it must be used with care and sensitivity. Unfortunately, many of us have come to mistrust praise, to feel that it is not genuine and hence to lose the value of its guidance. If a person feels good about something he has done, then praise feels good and encourages that behavior. If the person is very uncertain or negative about his own behavior, then outside praise is less effective.

The very best way to discover what to praise about your wife's behavior, and when to praise it, would be to try eating her diet yourself for several days, even if you are not actually trying to slim as well.

This will help you to know how it feels to live on a reduced food intake and tolerate a certain amount of deprivation. It may also give you a new respect for the job your wife is undertaking and for the strength she is already exhibiting.

What it should certainly do is make it clear that a weekly "round of applause" when your wife declares her weight loss is not all that is called for in the way of praise. All of us need more immediate "feed-back" to reassure us that we are on the right track and doing the things that will lead to long-term success. A person living in the same household is in the unique position of being able to note and praise all those very small but definite actions that lead to the end goal.

Just preparing that single meal, accurately and within correct dieting requirements, can be noted with approval. So can leaving a small portion of food on the plate, saying "No thank you" to food offered by others, and her controlled response to food and drink during a social occasion. Or even just the fact that she has gone through the evening without eating any of her usual extra snacks. Positive new ways of behavior relating to food control are just as important and praise-worthy as the restrictions of old eating patterns—the positive act that it takes to join and regularly attend a Slimming Club, embark on a daily program of exercise, or become involved in a new activity.

Remember that praise is not only verbal. A smile, a touch, a hug, can often convey loving approval more effectively than words. A side-benefit of this approach will be to reassure your wife that your love and her basic attractiveness are not dependent on her weight.

Your desire for her to lose weight must be seen as a desire for an improvement in a person you already find attractive, if it's to be a help rather than a direct hindrance to her slimming efforts.

Of course, the tool of praise is going to be of no use at all on those occasions when your wife does break her diet and succumbs to temptation. So, as criticism is detrimental, what can you do?

If you see her overeating, the best thing to do is to focus on her feelings rather than the eating itself. Often, the most effective approach is the direct one. Simply ask: "What's bothering you?"

While you don't want to be overbearing, you may have to be a bit persistent in getting her to talk to you about how she feels. Be a receptive and sympathetic listener, but don't feel you have to solve her problems. You might ask whether there is anything you can do to help her to feel better, but just listening will be the greatest help.

As she sees that you are a sympathetic listener, it will become easier for her to share these feelings with you, even before they lead to overeating. As a general rule it is often helpful to get a troubled person active after a period of tense worrying; active perhaps in solving a problem but, generally, any kind of activity helps. Sometimes, just getting out for a walk is a great boost.

It may be that you too have a weight problem—in which case, dieting together can be mutually helpful, but you should be aware of some possible pitfalls. You can praise and support one another for sticking to a diet; but if one member of the couple slips, it is all too easy for the other to support the idea of their both abandoning the diet. That is one of the reasons why a "slimming group" has advantages over a "slimming pair." Another problem to look out for, in a slimming twosome, is the adverse effect of competition. Often competition is helpful, but between two people it can sometimes hurt the loser more than it helps the winner. This is especially a problem for the wife, since men tend to lose weight more quickly and easily than women. The best remedy for these problems is open discussion and planning by the couple. Being alert to the pitfalls may be all that is necessary to avoid them.

Although this letter is addressed to the husband who wants to help his wife to become slim, one problem—which need not be serious—crops up often enough to be worthy of mention.

Some men are afraid of their wives' becoming really slim. They want them to be more attractive, yet when that begins to happen, particularly as the weight loss becomes obvious, they realize that the attractiveness may not be limited to their own eyes; their wives may be attractive to others as well as themselves.

I know of no statistics about the frequency with which formerly fat wives abandon their husbands, but I doubt whether the number is very large. Nevertheless, statistical reassurance is probably not very effective for most husbands. The best remedy to this problem lies in a wife's own hands. If she finds that her husband begins to sabotage her diet, especially after having supported her efforts, she should consider whether he is concerned about the danger of her new attractiveness. She will need to decide the best way to reassure him of his own attractiveness to her, by her words, attentiveness, and attitude. In the end, his reassurance may have to come from his wife sticking to her diet *and* to him.

The husband who really wants his wife to become slim can do very much more than he probably imagines he can to achieve his object.

But sensitivity and imagination are essential, so he must quickly discover that the proverbial *carrot* is the best of all—that the most dangerous and least helpful is the proverbial *stick*.

Yours sincerely,

chapter fifteen
UNDERASSERTIVENESS AND OVEREATING

"*No!*" That is one of the most useful and essential words in our vocabulary, but I wonder how much you have used it during the past few years. Probably, if you are overweight, you have a tendency to go along with other people's plans and wishes. You're the giver, the nice guy or girl who finds it hard to refuse. . . . Now there is nothing at all wrong with being "the nice guy"; being agreeable for the right reasons is a positive and pleasurable thing. But where it can go sour on you is when you say yes when you really want to say no. Then you start brooding about it and building up hostilities, and from there it's a very short step to the cookie jar. Let's take a hypothetical situation. Your next-door neighbor has started taking it for granted that she can park her children with you any time she chooses, and you are beginning to feel a little resentful of her casual attitude and all the inconvenience involved. But you don't *really* like to say anything. So the situation continues, and you begin to feel more and more resentful. You brood over the fact that she "imposed on you." You tell yourself that everyone else takes you for granted too.

Yet you continue to say nothing, and let that frustration build up to real anger; then maybe one day it all explodes and you say to her, furiously, "Look after your own kids!"

That isn't being an assertive person. The art of being assertive lies in being able to get what you need from your relationships with other people, without building up hostility and without having to resort to aggressiveness.

What has all this to do with your weight problem? Well, if you look for a direct link you will probably realize that when you fly to the comfort of the cookie jar you are often feeling hurt, frustration, taken for granted, or misunderstood. Overweight-prone people who see a psychological basis to their problem are inclined to explain their urge to overeat as being simply due to a lack of willpower. Actually, as we have seen, the problem is likely to be somewhat more complex—and like all psychological problems, this has much to do with relationships with other people, ranging right from the closest member of the family to the most casual acquaintances.

Your relationships with other people play a key part in weight control. And it is quite possible to change your personal relationships by learning to be a more assertive person.

Let's start by looking back to that hypothetical situation and considering why you allowed your neighbor to take advantage of you in the first place.

For the person who is sensitive about being overweight, the tendency to be agreeable has often developed as a defense mechanism, a kind of psychological protection policy. If, deep down inside, your excess weight has made you feel vulnerable—a possible object of ridicule—then it may feel essential to you that the other person should see you as the nice guy.

Otherwise, she may notice that you are fat. . . .

Otherwise, horror or horrors, she may even attack you and ridicule you in this area in which you feel you are totally defenseless.

But, as a protection policy against this vulnerability, the policy of always being the nice person is doomed to failure on many counts. Human relationships rarely work on a bank-account system; if conflicts arise, you can't rely on being able to draw on a store of goodwill. If a person wants to hurt you, the chances are that he or she is going to hurt you whatever you have done earlier. And by living in a constant state of retreat from conflict with other people, you are building up the much more damaging conflicts that go on inside yourself.

Paradoxically, the more easily you are able to say no, the less often you have to say it. If you are firm and say no when you really mean no and yes when you really mean yes, people will respect you in the way that they don't respect the nice guy.

In learning to be more assertive, you need to work at developing the two sides of this particular quality. You need to practice *positive assertiveness*, which has to do with going ahead and getting what you want out of life from others (this needn't be selfish, because it enables you to give to others in a more genuine way in return). And you also need to practice *negative assertiveness*, which prevents getting what you don't want, without the need for aggression or hostility.

We'll consider the negative assertiveness first, because this has more to do with the typical situation of the neighbor to which we have already referred. The primary error made by the "victim" lay in not taking some assertive action the moment she felt that her neighbor was beginning to take advantage of her. In any situation of this kind, waiting is usually an error. If you don't want to do something, the sooner you say so the better. The longer you wait, the more your tensions build up, and the more difficult it becomes to solve the situation without hostility.

Of course, the put-upon person could try to extricate herself by making excuses for not having her neighbor's children, but the pitfall of polite excuses is that they tend not to get us out of the trap. Often they have to be made over and over again before the message sinks in.

On the whole, we are inclined to underestimate the ability of other people to accept our assertiveness. Most people can take an honest and simple NO *without being alienated—without, at least, being alienated permanently.*

Honesty is usually the best policy. But the majority of us tend to overexplain ourselves, and the more we explain, the more dishonest we get: "No." "No—sorry!" "No—sorry, I can't because . . ."

With each added word, we are getting further away from the simple, basic truth. In this we are not suggesting just a blunt "No"—which can indeed be unnecessarily rude—in response to every unwelcome request. But it is important to resist the impulse to ramble on into paragraphs of explanation.

"The earlier the better" is the best rule for using assertiveness in all kinds of situations. The more you can anticipate people trying to take advantage of you, the better—and the earlier you make it clear that you are not going to be taken advantage of, the better.

Take the problem of the persistent sponger who always seems to succeed in leaving you to pay the bill. An early and direct assertive approach from you need not lead to any hard feelings.

"I'll pay for this drink—then let's go Dutch" or "I'll get the movie tickets this week, and you get them next week" can make your intentions quite clear without spoiling a friendship.

Or take the problem of the person who always wants you to shop for her but doesn't seem too willing to return the favor. The only way to prevent this from developing into a real cause of annoyance is to make it quite clear that you are doing this only as a part of a reciprocal arrangement: "Yes—I'd be glad to, if you will take care of such and such for me next week".

In these situations you can be assertive, with tact, and you'll usually succeed. But sometimes you may find that you have to be more bluntly direct and simply say, for instance: "No—it's your turn to pay the bill."

This isn't easy, so it's a good idea to practice being assertive in simple situations at first—for instance, when your friend suggests that you go to see a particular movie while you are really longing to see a different movie! It is really much better to say "No—I'd much rather go to this other movie," and then work out the problem in the open, then to spend an unenjoyable evening and come home with a smoldering feeling of resentment toward your friend. Even less easy is the problem of asserting yourself in public situations. For the person having difficulty being assertive, one of the most difficult people to deal with is often the power-deluded employee. We have all come across this person many times: the doctor's receptionist, the waiter in an expensive restaurant, the clerk in an elegant dress shop, the person you have to speak to over the desk in a government office.

It is very easy for people in jobs like these to take advantage of their situation if they're so inclined—because, unthinkingly, we tend to respond to them as if they had the authority and status of the power structures for which they merely work. Often it is necessary to remind ourselves that the waiter is just a waiter, however lavish and awe-inspiring the restaurant in which he works. Having gotten his job into perspective, it becomes easier to say, preferably with a smile: "No, this isn't what I ordered. Would you please bring me *broiled*, not fried, fish?"

To get what you want, it isn't necessary to become loud and complaining—because a problem dealt with swiftly, quietly, and assertively usually doesn't blow up into a major battle or scene.

Nevertheless, when you start asserting yourself in public, you are taking a chance. Standing up for yourself will not be easy, and some situations might prove too threatening and frightening. This fear has probably been affecting your relationships for a long time. So, let's look this problem straight in the eye. Imagine that, just on one occasion, your assertiveness leads to a direct clash. Let's say the person you are dealing with responds aggressively. What is worse, that person is vicious enough to attack you on your weakest and most vulnerable point.

Think of the worst thing he or she can say: you aren't just called a "so-and-so"—you are called a *"big fat* so-and-so"! What are you to say, think, and do?

We would suggest that one thing to do is to look at the person in blank astonishment and say, "I don't see what my weight has to do with what we are talking about. . . ." Maybe you can think up a better phrase, but the important thing is to face this as a possibility rather than leaving it as an unmentionable, irrational fear. This way you lose your fear of "the unknown," and by preplanning your response to the situation you gain confidence. You can think it through and leave it without becoming preoccupied and worrying in an unproductive way.

Whatever you say, it is still likely that you are going to feel somewhat distressed by this sort of situation, if it does arise. Even if you lose one skirmish, it is well worth the risk. For if we let our vulnerability prevent us from asserting our own personalities, we lose *every* time.

You know from bitter experience that every time you let a situation go by where you don't speak up for yourself, you invite a later postmortem examination—a trial in which you convict yourself for being spineless, cowardly, a failure, and so on. Similarly, if the anger aroused in you for doing something you didn't want to do for someone else never gets expressed, it eventually turns inward and is converted to self-criticism. The next step is eating.

If someone is constantly teasing you about your weight, you have probably tried laughing, appearing not to care, or even avoiding that person. But have you ever tried saying simply: "I find that remark very hurtful"?

Try it. You will probably be surprised at the effectiveness of the simple truth. Most people will sympathize with and respond to honest hurt.

It is equally important to be able to respond in the right way when something nice has been said to us. So often we feel uncomfortable when complimented, and argue the compliment away in a manner that will reduce the real benefit it can give to our self-evaluation.

All we need really say is: "Thank you, that makes me feel very nice." And once we become able to accept compliments, we become more able to see ourselves positively. Constantly tearing yourself down, constantly finding fault with yourself, constantly looking at the negative side is part of the problem that says "I'm not worth nice things—I'm fat." Some of the suggestions made so far may have led you to believe that we are advocating a very selfish and premeditated approach to life. This is not so. What matters is *why* you give help.

If you do a kindness for someone else willingly, happily, and because you *really* want to help, this will make you feel good and will increase your own self-evaluation. If, on the other hand, you do it grudgingly with the mistaken idea that if you're nice to them they'll be nice to you, you will be aware of your real motives, and this will decrease your self-evaluation.

You will find that people tend to place just as much value on you as you place on yourself.

Of course, there are situations where we make a rational, sometimes moral decision to put others ahead of ourselves. The suggestions given here are not directed to that sort of clear-cut choice, but to the tendency in many of us—out of our own insecurity—to extend this moral sphere inappropriately to a way of life that too often makes our own needs and desires a poor second. This tendency not only hurts us, but those around us, in the end. A difficult but common example is the parent who attempts to be the good father or mother by attending to the needs of the child regardless of his or her own current state of mind or body. Children, perhaps even more than adults, are sensitive to the resentment hidden behind attention or affection given more out of responsibility than from a genuine sense of wanting to give at the moment. Children get more from an hour of real time from a parent than from a whole day of dutiful attention.

To practice positive assertion, you need to consider what you need out of life and what you need from other people. Then you need to consider a simple step you probably haven't tried before: just asking for what you want.

This isn't always easy, particularly for the overweight person, because asking for help or cooperation usually involves a certain amount of self-disclosure. To some extent you have to reveal what is going on within you.

One specific issue that the person with a weight problem has to come to terms with, for instance, is how much she is willing to disclose about her eating problem.

Many people quite rightly regard what they eat as their own personal affair, something they don't have to explain to anyone. On the other hand, it is quite unrealistic to expect anyone else to be able to help you with this or any other problem unless he or she is aware of the problem's true nature.

It would be unrealistic to suggest that you have only to ask and everyone around you will respond to your every wish. But it is even more unrealistic to expect people to respond to your needs when they don't know what they are! So by asking—whether it is for cooperation, advice, help, or sympathy or affection in a love relationship—you are always increasing your chances of overcoming difficulties and frustrations.

It isn't possible to change overnight, but you can gradually learn to be a more assertive person. Start by making minor changes in areas where change might be a little difficult, but not overwhelmingly so. Having taken one small step, you are on your way. Feel free to refuse as well as to initiate; practice saying no when the occasion calls for it, even if at first it seems somewhat contrived. Don't let the distance from the ultimate goal stand in the way of the good feelings you can derive from each small success. The more you put yourself first in this special sense and start to live life your way, the more free you will be from these smoldering frustrations that tend to be confused with the sensations of hunger—and the less you will need to use food as a tranquilizer. The more you value yourself, the more you will value a slim body.

As with many other areas of self-change, the first step is analysis and planning. Make a list of your own problems in being assertive. The list can include a whole range of situations—some difficult and important, some relatively minor (for example, telling your husband you want his help around the house, asking your boss for a raise, keeping a waitress from serving you incorrectly, getting out of a project or work assignment, and so on). Next, order the list with numbers as to degree of difficulty for you—give the least difficult a 1, the next a 2, and so on. Begin with the number 1. Write it at the top of a blank sheet of paper. Beneath the statement of the situation, write out a strategy for being more assertive. Try to think of the easiest step first and then more difficult steps to take. This week take the first step toward being more assertive in situation number one, if it arises. If possible, get a friend or relative to help you in advance by rehearsing with you. Tell your friend about the situation and what you plan; then actually say the words you would want to say. Treat the sheet as a self-plan, giving yourself points or some definite reward for taking a new step. How do you know if you've been more assertive and deserve a point? As much as possible, the standard for self-reward should be your own judgment about your actual performance—not how comfortable you feel when you did it or even whether you succeeded, but just how well you feel you asserted yourself. Feeling at ease and gaining success takes time and will come as you practice. For example, we did some research on shy young college men who had difficulty in dating relationships. The situation to be dealt with was, "Asking a new girl for a date." We told the men to write out a sketch of what they would like to say on the phone and to give self-rewards just for doing that—*not* if it were done without feeling anxious; *not* if the girl accepted the date. *The main standard was each man's judgment about his own performance.*

Let's analyze an example having to do with assertiveness in

an eating situation. You are invited to a dinner party by an acquaintance (not a close friend) who is well known for her baking of elaborate, high-calorie desserts. Step one involves determining your own goal. Do you want to refuse the dessert? Do you want to ask for a very small portion? Do you want to take a normal portion, but eat only part of it? Whichever your goal, we'll assume you have planned for a given number of calories to be allowed for that evening. Perhaps you've reserved some calories by eating lightly that day (not by starving yourself beforehand).

In planning a strategy, several principles are helpful. First, remember that time can be your ally. The earlier you deal with the problem, the easier it will be. In this situation it's much easier to say at the time of *invitation*, "I'd love to come, but I want you to know I'm dieting and will need your help with getting small portions. Your pastries are fantastic, and I'll save up some calories for that night, but I hope you'll understand if I take a small amount." By doing it in advance you defuse the situation and have a better chance of getting what you want without offending the other person. If you choose to reveal the reason why you won't be taking certain foods, or will be taking small quantities, or even leaving food on your plate, you may be able to get the hostess's sympathy and cooperation. However, you may choose not to discuss your weight and to simply say that you are unable to eat certain foods. You can also make it clear that you don't want to discuss your diet at the party.

You need not be aggressive or hostile to be assertive. You can be gentle, light, even humorous in getting your point across. It's almost always possible to compliment the other person and get him on your side, especially if you give him or her time and opportunity to be helpful. Faced with a guest who leaves half a pastry, the hostess will be much more accepting of your compliments about her baking if she knows in advance what is going on. In preparing to be assertive in a situation, it's important to anticipate needing a second or even a third response. For example, if you say simply, "No, thank you" to the pastries, the hostess may say, "Oh, come on, they're my special recipe." You should then be prepared to respond with something like, "I know they're fantastic, but I must stick to my diet" (or, "They look wonderful, but I just can't"). But suppose she persists with, "I'll really be hurt if you don't even taste them." You could say, "Please don't be insulted; the dinner was superb, but my doctor won't permit me to eat sweets." Or, "You can't imagine how tempted I am, but I've got to keep up my willpower." You can see that there are many possible responses. The best approach is your own, and planning and rehearsing until you get the hang of it will help a lot.

During this week you should list several situations in your life that you feel require more assertiveness on your part. This could be done in conjunction with Chapter 14 on the family, focusing on assertiveness with someone who lives with you. Or you can emphasize assertion problems outside your home. Select any one of these situations, perhaps starting with one somewhat less difficult than the others, and write a detailed strategy for increasing your assertiveness gradually. Then during this week begin to practice being more assertive in that type of situation.

To help you further, here is another example of assertion strategy.

The situation: Whenever a certain friend or relative (spouse, parent, etc.) comes to your house, he or she brings along some high-calorie food to share with you. For example, a husband brings home doughnuts; a mother brings a "CARE" package of her homemade baked goodies; a friend comes over for coffee and brings pastries.

Overall Goal: Your overall goal is to stop the person from doing this. You must first decide how important it is to stop it without damaging the relationship with that person. That is, how blunt and direct can you be with this person?

For example, your spouse brings home doughnuts (or ice cream, etc.) It appears that he or she is doing this as a way of being nice, of giving me a gift that he thinks I will like. Therefore, your goal might be to get him to show his affection in other ways.

The preceding example, by using positive means and understanding, shows success in rechanneling other people's behavior. In some situations this constructive approach doesn't seem to work. The other person persists. You then face the choice of avoiding that person (or that person in that situation) or increasing your assertion. This means saying what you want stronger and/or louder. For example, "I will not be able to see you if you keep bringing these foods." Or, "You are sabotaging my efforts to control my eating. This has got to stop." There are many possible responses. While it is difficult, the only way to do it is to practice and gradually face these kinds of situations.

During the next few weeks, continue to rehease your strategy for the first situation sheet and work your way step by step toward your goal of assertiveness in that type of situation. Remember that you should reward yourself for taking each step. *Don't worry about whether you felt uncomfortable trying and don't penalize yourself if your efforts didn't get you what you set out for.* The main thing is to reward yourself for trying. You can also begin working on the other situations as you begin to feel some confidence about your improvement in the first type of assertion situation.

This chapter on assertion has focused, naturally enough, on being more assertive with people. As a final note, be aware that assertiveness involves dialogue, and that some of your most important dialogue is with yourself. All of us talk to ourselves (though most do it quietly enough so as not to be labeled crazy). We talk most about problem areas. Overweight people talk about eating and food—especially trying to control mis-eating—by talking to themselves as a parent talks to a child. A colleague psychologist has suggested that you can train yourself to be more assertive with someone else by practicing new dialogues. One way to do this is to put the dialogue outside. That is, instead of talking to another part of yourself, talk to the food; this not only increases aware eating, as we suggested in Chapter 5, but it improves assertiveness. Try sentences like: "You're not going to push me around," "I'll eat you if *I* want to, not just because you look so appealing." You can shout and scream at the food if no one is around to hear you. If you get really angry at a particular food for tempting you, smash it with your fist, or even stomp on it with your feet. All of this may sound a bit far out, but consider it as a fun experiment which may turn out to be very useful.

SUGGESTED PARTNER ACTIVITY

When you have read this chapter on assertiveness, you will realize that there are three areas in which you can be of help to your partner:

1. Helping her to be more assertive in her relationships with others.
2. Being more assertive yourself and providing a model for her.
3. Helping both of you to understand and clarify assertion issues between the two of you.

There are several ways you can help your partner improve her assertion with others. You can discuss the problem areas and help her set up her plan. You can set up a rehearsal in which you play the parts of people she wants to be assertive toward, or you can play her part to show her how you would do it. You should proceed very carefully with this kind of help, doing only as much as your partner wants from you. If you do rehearse with her, try to help her proceed slowly. Try to be as patient as possible with her. And, of course, help her with the setting up of rewards for her achievements in the steps of her plan.

If you decide to practice improving your own assertion, it is important that you try to establish a reciprocal helping relationship with your partner. Let her help you in the same ways that you help her. Sometimes helping another person is a great way to improve yourself.

Assertion issues between you and your partner could provide material for a whole book in itself. Questions of power in a relationship range from the trivial (who does the dishes) to the vital (how financial decisions are made, or who initiates sex). The two of you will have to decide whether this is a time in your relationship when you want to discuss issues of assertion between you. It is a difficult area, and you need not feel guilty if you say, "Let's leave this box closed for a while." If you decide to work on a particular area, you may want to get outside help from a professional counselor. The rehearsal technique is awkward when you are the real person she wants to assert toward. So the only practical help you can give, without an outside counselor, is to be open to discussion and negotiations on assertion issues that your partner may wish to raise.

chapter sixteen
SCARED TO BE SLIM

Jim had been sixty pounds overweight and lost the weight quickly on a near-total fast. He weighed less than he had weighed since high school and was enjoying compliments from all sides. In fact, some people commented that he looked too thin. He found himself tense at meals, almost afraid to eat, and was thinking about the possibility of setting a new goal five pounds lower.

There is an obstacle, a wall that often arises near the end of dieting. It usually appears at a stage when there is sufficient change in your looks and self-image for people to start reacting to you differently. Yes, we appreciate that since you so loathed being overweight it was very hard for you to imagine that you could possibly ever have any reaction against the idea of being thin. However, this is in fact a very common experience, particularly among those who have been seriously overweight. If you go around the wall without conquering it, the bar of being slim will plague you and send you back up the weight-gain path.

The fact is that unpleasant though it is in so many ways, there are actually some payoffs in being overweight. It lets you off the hook in some respects. Weight can be used as an excuse for delaying positive acts that demand some effort. For instance, the bored overweight housewife who has been saying for years she must get a job has been adding "as soon as I lose this weight."

Now, as she sees the first positive signs that she is getting slim, she has to face the fact that she is also losing her reason for delaying taking a step which, understandably, she really views with a certain amount of hesitation and trepidation.

For a person who has been sufficiently overweight to have lost her femininity to some extent there is the sudden awareness that she now has to make the effort to be feminine. The same holds true for men, though masculinity is less talked about in our culture. Often, as her (his) size decreases, the first compliment she receives reawakens something in her mind. Over the years she may gradually have opted out of making the effort to be feminine—not specifically in the sexual sense, but in her social role and in her appearance. Her relationships with other women have developed on a comfortable, noncompetitive basis. There is no doubt that her change in weight is likely to change the basis of these relationships. There is something in all of us, too, that makes us like to be noticed—and surplus weight can attract attention, even though it is usually attention of the least welcome kind. There was one very overweight woman in a group who used to refer to herself as "a monstrosity," but who nevertheless enjoyed dancing and boasted that she was still light on her feet.

It was clear that she stood out in a crowd, that her physical size gave her some sort of status. We don't want to belittle the fact that she was hurt over and over again—but she was noticed. Very often such fears are vague and not much thought about, but they can lead to sufficient conflict to make a slimming effort fizzle out.

There are many people who will tell you that they seem to have a weight-loss barrier: "I can never seem to get below 140. . . . " That barrier will often be located at a weight where they have ceased to be very overweight and are just approaching becoming slim.

There can be straightforward dieting reasons for this barrier; sometimes a stricter diet might be needed for continued weight loss at this stage. But the kind of psychological reasons we have described can be a major factor in erecting this barrier, and usually people are not really aware of what it is that is keeping them from their goal. A realistic self-assessment is the essential first step needed to overcome this type of obstacle. Once you can say "I'm scared," and figure out what you are scared of, you take a big step forward. You can now say, "What can I do about it?" You can decide either to do something directly about it or you can make up your mind to tolerate the fear until you begin to experience some of the positive benefits of being slim.

THE FEAR OF REGAINING WEIGHT.   This is a very real fear that will be experienced by the majority of slimmers once they reach their target weight. It can even occur—and put an end to slimming —before the goal is reached. The feeling, illogical as it sounds, is that it is better to fail now than to achieve the goal and then lose it. *That* would be really terrible. . . .

The important thing about this fear of regaining weight is that a certain amount of it is good and realistic. If you held no fears of this nature, you might well regain weight. On the other hand, your fear should not be so great as to throw you into a state of panic. Too much of any fear can be an obstacle to staying slim.

To avoid this panic level, you need to learn to be realistic. It is unrealistic to imagine that once you are slim, no more moments of stress will arise. Accept the fact that resorting to comfort eating from time to time, at times of stress, is not a total disaster that cancels out all other efforts you make at weight control.

We all have to expect failure and learn how to cope with it, whether it is a brief failure or a longer one which will cause your weight to increase.

Basically, it is a very sound idea for every successful slimmer to set herself a maximum weight slightly higher than goal weight, which allows for a modest degree of failure. Set yourself a "safe-range" limit. Agree on a weight—perhaps write it on the scale—a few pounds over the target weight you achieved. This way, modest gains within the safe-range limit can be corrected without your getting any feeling of panic. Concentrate on catching them and correcting them as quickly as possible. While some ex-slimmers regain weight very rapidly, most receive ample warning that corrective action needs to be taken.

For many people, the fear of regaining weight revolves

around the fear they have of being unable to control their desire for certain foods. They will tell you, "Once I start eating chocolate, I'm lost. . . . "

Any slimmer who has completely eliminated these foods from her menu during her period of dieting has good reason to be afraid, because it is unlikely that she is going to resist these particular foods forevermore. And once she succumbs to "a bite," she has no self-control training in this area to stop a bite from leading to a binge, just as it always used to do before.

That is why we recommend that high-temptation foods should be introduced into a slimming program at some stage. By practicing the methods we have taught in Chapter Eleven—first making sure that only a small quantity of the temptation food is available to be eaten, then gradually progressing to the stage where you eat a little and are able to leave the rest of it—you will find that you cope with the maintenance period of weight control with a great deal more confidence.

You will have made a deliberate change. You will have already put in a good deal of the practice and training that is necessary to gain self-control over your high-termptation foods.

THE FEAR OF LOOKING LIKE A FOOL.   Suppose you have carefully set yourself a safe-range limit. Then, perhaps during a somewhat trying period in your personal life, you find your weight rising above that carefully marked line on the scales. It can happen. And it can feel very bad: "I'm failing, I'm slipping back. . . ." The panic sets in. And the more you panic, the more guilty you feel, the more you lose control.

This feeling of guilt at a setback is a major obstacle to permanent weight control. It is a very automatic and widespread reaction that you must guard against.

Before becoming slim, you had probably labeled yourself as a fat failure; unfortunately, your self-image usually doesn't change as quickly as your weight. For some time you continue to think of yourself as a fat person "masquerading" as a slim person. Therefore it is easy to think, as you start to regain weight, that the real truth is re-emerging, inevitably and hopelessly.

Yet, usually you will begin to feel this sense of demoralizing shame before anyone else even notices that you are regaining weight.

To overcome this obstacle and get hold of the situation, you are going to have to face some realistic facts about yourself and about life in general.

Life doesn't stay the same; we are all put under some stresses from time to time. And when faced with stress, the majority of people tend to turn to the comfort of some form of overindulgence, whether it is smoking, drinking, sex, or, in your case, mis-eating. Some people will suffer from ulcers, some from headaches; your past experience will show that when life becomes difficult your pattern is to gain weight.

By looking at it in this way, you will see that regaining weight need be no more shaming than suffering from an ulcer. The person suffering from an ulcer will go on a controlled eating plan to correct the problem. In the same way, you need to go back on more controlled intake to correct your problem.

You are going to have to admit to some people that you are back in training again.

You aren't a failure *unless* you fail to face up to the problem and take the necessary steps required at this stage. You should just regard this as another move forward in the process of successfully learning control. One of the attitudes common to many overweight people involves seeming themselves as all bad or all good. Such a perfectionist policy demands that you either succeed 100 percent in eating control, all the time, or you consider yourself "off the wagon" and back again in the failure syndrome. Any form of rigid self-labeling ("I am obese," "I am a bad person," "I am weak-willed," or even "I am good") can get in the way of efforts to change. This view has to be replaced by a realistic policy that allows for limited degrees of failure followed by positive and confident steps to correct that temporary failure.

You have, in fact, achieved marked progress—scored a real success—if you catch that weight gain and start to tackle it again before it rises to those previous proportions. That is an encouraging sign of change. It shows you are moving forward.

THE LOSS OF A GOAL.   For real satisfaction, all human beings need to have a feeling that they are moving forward, growing, progressing—and this brings us to another of the unexpected obstacles you will face after reaching your target weight.

You have gotten what you wanted—but you have lost a goal.

In most of life's situations, it is hard to grade success. But not in slimming. Your weekly weight losses give you a continual flow of tangible rewards for your efforts.

After slimming there will be the rewards of the compliments and all the positive benefits you receive, but you may miss the actual feeling of moving forward in a purposeful direction.

To consolidate your weight loss it will help if, at this stage, you look at the options now open to you and embark on some new interest or project. The person you were when you were overweight may have lacked sufficient absorbing interests and goals in life. The new person you are becoming needs to consider how he or she can continue to develop and use newfound confidence in other directions. And this change, with its continuing feeling of psychological growth, will do much to make your change in shape become permanent.

THE MIRACLES THAT DON'T HAPPEN.   Many people embark on a slimming campaign with the idea that it will solve *all* life's problems. A great deal does happen, many problems are solved, and we have yet to meet a successful slimmer who said it wasn't worth the effort.

However, let's look at the situation of, say, the divorced woman who has embarked on a slimming campaign in the hope that once she has gotten slim another potential husband will appear.

It is quite true that becoming slim and more attractive will be of great benefit to her in finding another husband. But she might get slim and then find that the miracle doesn't necessarily happen right away.

There is a great tendency here to feel let down. And a danger that she might tell herself, "Well, it didn't work, so I might as well go back to food." Or take the case of the wife who is very dissatisfied with her marriage. Often, because of her increased confidence in herself, enough happens after a successful slimming campaign to set the process of improvement under way.

Again, though, we have to consider the realistic fact that the root cause of the marriage problem may have been her husband's problem—not her weight at all. Many a woman reports a gratifying change in her husband's attitude after she has lost weight: "He doesn't take me for granted any more." But if the husband is bad-tempered, inattentive, and difficult to live with mainly because of problems he is experiencing at work, it would be unrealistic to expect his wife's weight change to provide a total cure for marriage problems.

In these sorts of situations, it is important to face up to things in a positive way and consider the steps that are now open to you. You have solved your weight problem; what are the ways in which you can solve your other problems, too?

First of all, sit down and look at those photographs of yourself as you were when you were fat, and remind yourself of all the things you hated about being fat. You may have to do this reasonably frequently to remind yourself that getting fat again won't solve any problems at all, that it will only add to them.

Your main asset lies in self-awareness that you can overcome a problem—your weight problem—which at one time seemed extremely difficult to impossible to solve. You can, in a similar way, begin to solve other problems which also seem to be almost insurmountable.

Ultimately, everyone—whatever their situation—has to rely upon themselves to make their own lives interesting and rewarding; getting slim should just be regarded as the first big step that will make that process possible. Slimming is not an end in itself. By making yourself take other first steps, often in directions you may never have considered before, you can make important changes happen. Perhaps the miracle won't be quite as you envisaged it at first. Who knows, possibly it will be even better.

Whether you are near your goal weight or still have a distance to go, it would be helpful to anticipate some of your personal obstacles to weight maintenance. Prepare a list of these, and next to each jot down a few ideas about how you might overcome that obstacle when or if it appears.

When you have reached your goal weight and felt comfortable with it for at least a month, try a *planned relapse*. Instead of waiting, dreading the first time the scale will go back up, make it happen on purpose. Select a time period when you think your life will be relatively calm and intentionally gain three or four pounds. Write down how you feel as it's happening, any guilt or fears that crop up. Note how you chose to add weight—what foods, what situations. If you're working with a partner, be sure to tell him/her what you're doing.

Plan your own recovery. Will you keep a diary? Go on a fast or diet? Increase your physical exercise? How quickly will you take the weight back off?

When you reach your goal weight again, review the whole experience and decide whether you can use the same recovery strategy again, or whether you want to plan some other alternative. The important point of this exercise is to realize that you have learned a lot of self-control, that you can handle a relapse by catching it early and planning a recovery strategy.

SUGGESTED PARTNER ACTIVITY

If your partner stays with the principles of control we have communicated to her, she will approach her goal weight. Although it may not happen until sometime in the future, she may have her own fears about approaching goal weight; and you may have some of your own. Although this topic may not be relevant now, it may become very important when success comes near.

We know that you have positive feelings about your partner's approaching slimness. However, most partners tend to have mixed feelings. In one study, many men were asked what it would mean to them if their wives became slim. Many said they feared that their wives would be unfaithful and that they might lose them to divorce; others thought that they might lose some of their bargaining position in arguments. There may be some bases to these fears. Certainly, as your partner becomes more attractive to you, she will also become more attractive to others; and as she attains the confidence in herself that naturally results from a successful effort in self-control, she may be a better contender in an argument. These kinds of changes, however, need not seriously threaten your partnership.

This week we would like you to try to sort out what you think the consequences of your partner's approaching slimness might be. Take a sheet of paper and divide it into two columns. On one side, list all the positive things, and on the other, all the negative consequences of your partner's eventual slimness. The positive effects you list will be no problem to deal with. For the negative side, we can suggest to you the same thing we have suggested to your partner. The best thing to do is recognize what causes fear and apprehension for you and try to assess it realistically. If an anticipated negative consequence is not simply an unrealistic product of your imagination, you must decide what you need to do about it.

Once your partner attains goal weight, or even before, the issue of regaining the weight comes up. You have seen in this program how *active* the self-control process has to be. You have participated in many activities in our program that your partner has undertaken to take control of her eating. Activity is just as important in *weight maintenance*.

New activities or expanding present activities can help your partner stave off old eating habits if they begin to creep up. If you can support her approaches to new activities which keep her interests alive, this will help. Of course, you may not be totally comfortable having your partner invest her energies in new projects. It is a natural thing for one member of a couple to feel a sense of loss or anger when the other one moves in a different, self-determined direction. If you find yourself having this kind of reaction when your partner is marking new territory for herself, try to think what good it might bring her. In spite of initial negative reactions, if one member of a couple is doing his or herself some good, that person brings a more satisfied self back into the relationship. Both partners then benefit.

Another aspect of the issues we are discussing has to do with your partner's own difficulties in approaching activities and projects she avoided before she lost weight. If you notice signs of difficulty occurring as she approaches her goal weight, you should not be surprised. Your partner, in this case, has to deal with her own fears and apprehensions and decide how she is going to tackle them. As usual, you cannot do it for her, but you can help by lending a listening ear and offering thoughts you have that might help her see a route to solving her problems. Similarly, you should help your partner set up an early-warning system to pick up signs of weight regain, and then to reinstitute techniques (for example, diary keeping) that have helped her the most during this program.

Finally, the actual work on eating habits must continue for your partner to maintain her new slimmer status. The exercises you have practiced during the program will help your partner in the weight-maintenance period as they have in the weight-reduction period.

chapter seventeen
A METHOD FOR YOUR MADNESS

The most important message we can give you now is *Don't stop*! We've taught you a lot, but it's probably just beginning to sink in. It will take many weeks or months to reach a goal weight, get comfortable with new habits, and establish a workable maintenance pattern. There is a great tendency to use the ending of a program or a phase in a program as an excuse to stop working on your problem. Don't give in. Now is the time to really buckle down and work even harder.

This book did not provide you with a miracle cure, but perhaps it gave you some insights, changed some attitudes, and provided you with some strategies and skills to attack the multifaceted problem of weight control.

The next six months is critical in your efforts to achieve *permanent* weight control. You will have to take what we have provided and establish a pattern of self-control. We feel that the effectiveness of the methods we have presented lies in promoting independence from the start. You should continue many of the procedures given in the book and practice the critical skills until you become confident that they are second nature to you.

You will use some of the skills regularly, and some you will use periodically when the need arises. We will suggest a format for the next few months. It's important to remember that well-practiced techniques serve two purposes: 1) better day-to-day functioning of self-control and 2) a better chance to maintain all or part of your self-control in the face of crises. Stresses and emergencies will occur; they do for all of us. You are bound to see an increase in your eating, and a subsequent increase in weight, under such conditions. *Remember that the only failure is the failure to recover.* Your goal is to recoup your losses. Recognize your mistakes. Plan how to get back on the track, and do it.

At times of partial failure, what you say to yourself about yourself is critical. If you fall into the trap of labeling yourself as a failure, you will be more likely to grow to fit your own label. The secondary effects of being overweight are often worse than the weight itself. Labeling yourself as a failure, ugly, weak-willed, or any other negative image increases your negative feelings and pushes you to even more mis-eating. Accept yourself as basically okay and subject to human mistakes, and you'll be on your way to change.

Now let's look more concretely at a strategy for the next few months.

Daily Calorie Goal

It's vital that you continue to adjust your daily calorie goal. Until you have reached your goal weight and when you are not using a structured diet, you will want to have a calorie goal that will give you a gradual loss of one to two pounds per week. This figure will change for several reasons: Your weight is getting lower (it takes fewer calories of energy to maintain and move a smaller body), your extra physical activity level should be increasing (allowing for a slightly higher intake), and your metabolism may change. If you have gone two weeks without a weight loss, drop your goal by 100–200 calories (or increase your energy output). If you are at 1000 calories per day and not losing, try the following strategies: Check the accuracy of your portion judgment and calorie counting; shift to a greater proportion of protein over carbohydrate; increase physical exercise; try a one-day fast; check with your physician about fluid retention. Be sure to look at the day-to-day relationship of calories to weight. You may find a difference between the first and second half of the week (for example, a lower calorie total for three days, with a weight loss, then a slightly higher count and a gain). Examine why you changed midweek and set your goal at the first half-week's level.

When you reach your goal weight you cannot, of course, return to your old intake level. However, you can *gradually* increase your calories. Increase your daily calorie goal by 100 for a period of a week. If your weight stays steady, try another 100 for the next week. At some point you'll see an increase. Don't be frightened. Drop your goal back 100 at that point. Then try increasing about 100 again a week later. Perhaps your body will tolerate it now. If so, continue to increase. If not, you've probably found your steady state of calorie intake for that time. Stay at that level for several weeks. If it's comfortable, keep it permanently. If you'd like to try a higher level a month later, do so, but be prepared to drop back again if you see a gain in weight.

These calculations are based on your record keeping. When will you be able to stop keeping a food diary? Some of you will find, after several weeks at goal weight, that you are able to regulate your intake at the new level without a diary. You're knowledgeable about calories and portion size, and can have a feel for it without a written record. Others will have to continue keeping diaries for many months after reaching goal weight. (Everyone will need to keep diaries until *at least a month* after reaching goal weight). You can experiment with not keeping a diary for a week or two when things seem really settled and comfortable. Be prepared to return to diary keeping if trouble arises. Often, after a period of time at goal weight, people are able to use the scale to indicate the level of structure they need. They continue to weigh daily. If weight creeps up over a safety range (for example, five pounds over goal), they institute control measures, like diary keeping, until they're back below goal and stable again. Sometimes this swing is very regular; for example, free on weekends and strict calorie counting on weekdays. Each of you will work out your own level of structure when you reach that stage.

What About Diets?

We indicated early in the book that structured diets are sometimes useful, but are temporary tools. It does no good to go on and off diets to lose weight, without learning the kind of permanent system of self-control presented in this book. However, once you have learned such a system (or even while you are learning it), you may periodically use such techniques as diets or fasting. As long as you view these techniques as *temporary* aids in the context of long-term self-regulation, you will be able to return to the more permanent and hopefully more comfortable system we have been teaching you.

A BASIC LIST OF TECHNIQUES
FOR LONG-TERM SUCCESS

This book has crowded in a lot of information and techniques. You may find this a bit overwhelming and want a somewhat simpler structure for the coming months. We have selected what we feel are the most important methods and will summarize them briefly below.

1. *Food Diary.* You should by now have memorized the calorie values of the basic foods you eat regularly so that the diary is easy to keep. Periodically, you may have to look up an unusual food, but you should strive for independence. This also means being able to judge portion sizes consistently and also periodically testing your accuracy.

2. *Physical Activity.* You should be keeping your output up in three ways: by increasing output in daily activities (like climbing stairs instead of using elevators), by finding an enjoyable and regular form of physical recreation, and by walking regularly (especially after meals).

3. *Relaxation and Imagination.* You should have a regular time each day and a favorite method for physically and mentally relaxing. You can use this technique especially at times of stress. When

relaxed, you can use your imagination in many ways to improve self-control.

4. *Recognizing Hunger and Tolerating Delay.* You are better able to notice physical signs of real hunger, and you realize now that hunger need not be painful, that it waxes and wanes rather than growing steadily stronger. You can tolerate it for a while, especially if you can use various techniques (like physical activity) to distract yourself while you delay eating.

5. *Awareness of Emotions.* You are aware of the way other emotions get confused with real hunger. Recognizing emotions helps you to express them more directly, deal with causes for emotional upsets, and get emotional needs fulfilled more adequately. If you decide to eat for emotional reasons, your awareness helps you to eat the best foods in the best way.

6. *Eat in a Regular Place Without Distractions* (especially TV or reading). The general rule is to get the most mileage out of every bite. By focusing on your eating and really enjoying it, you can get more from less quantity. By eating in a regular place, you reduce the tendency to snack in an automatic and less-aware state of mind.

7. *Eat Slowly.* Eating slowly helps you to be aware physically of getting satisfied and aware mentally to make decisions about when to stop.

8. *Leave Food.* We taught you that you so often are served more than you need or want (if you're honest with yourself). Cleaning up your plate is wasteful in the long run because you ultimately eat so much more. Learning to stop is a vital part of self-control. Even high-temptation foods can be gradually brought under control so that you can eat small amounts with great satisfaction and stop.

9. *Planned, Constructive Mis-eating.* Sometimes none of the techniques of preventative action work completely, and you can decide to mis-eat. Then you can go about planning how to do this in a constructive way. An important element in doing this is to minimize guilt, which tends to lead to even more mis-eating. Each episode of mis-eating should end with an analysis of what happened and a plan for the future.

10. *Reading "Reasons to Lose Weight."* This list which you carry with you can be periodically revised as you see new and perhaps more important reasons. Reading the card can serve as a daily reminder and as a boost to your motivation at times when you feel pessimistic about your progress and your ability to proceed.

11. *Analyzing Problems and Writing Solutions.* We have emphasized a problem-solving approach to eating control. Your weight problem is in fact a series of problems which can be analyzed and alternative solutions planned. Having these written out and perhaps posted where you can see them will increase your chances of trying a new approach the next time the problem arises.

12. *Self-Plans and Rewards.* Carrying out a new solution can be facilitated by writing a personal plan that states the problem and the goal, lays out a series of steps to take, keeps a careful record of progress, and provides a concrete reward for completing the agreed actions. Giving yourself rewards and generally increasing pleasures in life while controlling eating should be an important element.

13. *Planned Assertiveness.* Increasing both positive assertion (getting what you want) and negative assertion (preventing others from taking advantage) is important in two ways: by controlling situations where your eating control is sabotaged, and by increasing your general sense of competence and thereby decreasing the frustration that leads to mis-eating. A planned program of increasing assertiveness with rehearsal and a personal plan can be a useful strategy.

Obviously, you will not use all of these techniques all of the time, but they are basic to your progress, and you should consider how to incorporate them into your day-to-day efforts. Items 4–8 comprise what we have called Aware Eating, which should increasingly replace uncontrolled eating as you gain competence in these skills.

14. *Involving Others and Getting Involved.* Continue to involve your family or any partners working with you on weight control. As you become more and more successful, look for ways to help others and to promote any successful techniques you've learned. In the past, some of our most ardent clients have organized discussion groups to help one another with weight control or maintenance.

TEST YOUR KNOWLEDGE

We have included in the Appendix a test of your knowledge of the material presented in the book. It's not a hard test, but is designed to show you how much you now know about your problem. More important, you now know what to do. Weight control is a difficult problem for millions of us. We hope that the material in this book helps you on your way to better control and a more pleasurable eating life-style. Best wishes for continuing success.

SUGGESTED PARTNER ACTIVITY

The same basic message that we give your partner at this point applies to you: *This is not the end.* You have worked hard, you understand your partner's task, and you know ways in which to help her. Whether she has reached her goal weight or has many pounds yet to lose, she will need your continued help and support for quite a while before she feels completely comfortable with handling mis-eating problems. Moreover, no matter how well a person has done, the future always brings times of stress and the threat of a new round of weight gain. So we hope that this program is a beginning for you both in the difficult but rewarding task of achieving a greater sense of self-control.

Just as we are listing the basic techniques for your partner in this final chapter, we would like to summarize the concepts and responses we have presented to you during the program. You may use all of them or only a few, but it is important for you to know the areas where you need to be alert and know the resources for change that are available to you.

1. *Reward.* We have urged you to focus your attention on the various behaviors that help your partner achieve control over eating, rather than emphasizing foods or quantities eaten. Find ways of rewarding her that are effective and genuine, whether they be verbal praise or physical reaching out. Use rewards frequently, but beware of trying to overcome your partner's own self-criticism. You may feel she has done something praiseworthy, but if she is self-critical, the compliment won't be heard. If you see this resis-

tance, pull back and ask her to set realistic goals in that area (for example, slow eating) so that next time you can both agree on what behavior can be rewarded.

2. *Avoid Nagging.* It is very difficult to be neutral, to see behavior you feel is negative and not only say nothing about it, but avoid nonverbal nagging (scrowls, heavy silence, etc.). Try to remember that your responsibility lies in the positive things summarized in this list, and not in being a policeman or parent for your partner. Discuss the areas in which you have done your nagging and tell your partner that you are trying to stop. She should be sympathetic with your efforts and with your occasional lapses. Try to lighten the situation and perhaps even joke a little about your own oral problems (over what comes out of rather than what goes into your mouth!).

3. *Help versus Independence.* Each of us has to come to terms with this conflict within ourselves. From the times as a child when we angrily said, "I'll do it myself," we have worked toward independence. Society values independence and criticizes excessive dependency in those not physically disabled. Yet we often go too far and, in stony silence, refuse to ask for help, attempting to hide every sign of weakness. This program has urged you to help your partner and urged her to recognize the need for help from you. But we have emphasized limiting that help to certain areas and continually recognizing the areas in which the person is moving toward self-control. There are no firm, universal rules for resolving this conflict, but know that the conflict is there and openly discuss areas where your partner wants more or less involvement from you; conversely, discuss areas where you may want to be more or less involved.

4. *Similarities and Differences Between Partners.* By recording your own food intake, activity, and weight for one week, you and your partner become aware of the differences between you in your energy balances. As the program has progressed, you should both have a better picture of your respective food requirements for losing or maintaining weight.

5. *Stress at the Table.* Perhaps just as difficult as inhibiting nagging is the task of inhibiting arguments and "negative vibes" at the

table. Creating a relaxed and pleasant atmosphere while eating can be a big challenge but a very worthwhile one to meet. If either of you is a person who mis-eats under stress, you don't want stress increased at the table. Look for the common causes of problems at meals and see if you can make a resolution to solve things in advance of eating or shelve them until afterward.

6. *Awareness of Your Mis-eating*. It has probably been a great relief for your partner to know that you, too, mis-eat, whether or not you have a weight problem, and that you really can share these problems and the search for solutions. Sharing with her how you react to stress and what coping methods you use may be the greatest benefit of this joint program.

7. *Mutual Pleasures List*. Eating is a pleasure, and we hope you both have found it even more so after this program. But we cannot stress too strongly the importance of alternative pleasures. Having pleasures that you share will further enhance your combined efforts in solving a whole range of problems.

8. *Knowing and Managing Your Eating Environment*. By now you should be very aware of where foods are stored and eaten in your home. You will have faced the issue of foods that are yours and, at least temporarily, not being eaten by your partner. It is hoped that these foods will be few and stored separately. You will know whether eating while watching TV (or at any other nonmeal time) is a problem for your partner, and you will have discussed how to handle these temptations to mis-eat.

9. *Grocery Shopping and Planning for Restaurant Meals or Parties*. You can assist your partner by occasionally shopping with her and encouraging her to use a shopping list. You can discuss restaurants, possible menus, and problems to be faced in advance of eating out. You can assist with parties by discussing ways to help your partner avoid mis-eating—not only during, but immediately before and after the party.

10. *Avoid Sabotage*. Whether consciously or unconsciously motivated, you may occasionally slip and bring your partner her favorite temptation food. Be aware that you can show your love in many ways and that the Valentine candy or surprise doughnuts may have to be permanently off limits in your family.

11. *Attitudes Toward Leaving Food.* Leaving food is one of the hardest tasks, and your partner may need your help to overcome old habits and the misconception that it is sinful not to clean her plate. If you can shift your own attitudes and even encourage your partner (and children, too) to waste a little, the payoff later will be far greater than the small loss now.

12. *Share Extra Physical Activities.* Getting into sports or even extra walking may be an obstacle for your partner. We have found that in the long run, this change may be even more important for permanent weight reduction than changes in food intake. As in so many areas, sharing the activity will make it more enjoyable and will provide frequent mutual reminders and rewards for participation. We are not suggesting competing with each other, but finding physical activities that are mutually pleasurable (in addition to sex).

13. *Model Slow and Sensual Eating.* We have suggested that you can be a great help by slowing down your own eating if it tends to be fast and by focusing both your and your partner's attention on the enjoyment of every bite of food.

14. *Company in the Kitchen.* Being alone while preparing or cleaning up may be a high-temptation time for your partner. If so, try to be with her as much as possible. You may or may not actually help with the work; division of household labor is a family matter. But even if you are not helping, you can simply be there or be doing some other activity in the area. This is not to create a surveillance system, but a support system, with conversation and even physical contact as a source of strength at a difficult time.

15. *Help With Relaxation.* If physical tension leading to mis-eating is a problem area for your spouse, the muscle relaxation exercise may be especially important for her. Set aside regular times to help her with this exercise, either by reading the instructions aloud or going through it together.

16. *Empathizing With Emotions.* We have suggested that you become more aware of your spouse's emotions, especially if they are not openly expressed and tend to lead to mis-eating. It's not your responsibility to solve the problem leading to the emotion, but to do everything you can to facilitate expression. A simple, "Do you want to talk about it?" may be all that's necessary.

17. *Sharing Binges.* When all else fails, your partner may experience the pressure to go on an all-out binge. Try to keep the channels of communication open about this so that she need not feel ashamed to admit what's happening. Plan the binge together in great detail, even writing a shopping list and menu. Share the cooking. Discuss every detail and encourage her to keep talking about her feelings, hunger sensations, and enjoyment of the food. Help her to minimize the guilt afterward, not by criticizing her expression of guilt, but by listening and then simply saying, "Let's plan how to tackle the problem next time."

18. *Encourage Assertiveness.* You may not want to turn your lamb into a lion, but after some difficult experiences of having her assert herself to you, you will also appreciate the sense of strength and confidence she has achieved. You can help her plan to be assertive with others, role play what she will say (with your taking the role of the opponent), and help her realistically evaluate herself afterward.

19. *Calm Your Fears About Partner's Becoming Slim.* All partners have mixed feelings about having a more attractive mate who also may be more attractive to others. Discuss your fears and ask for reassurance if necessary.

20. *Plan For Backsliding.* Know that your partner will some day regain weight. Discuss her being open with you about this. Agree on what amount of regain will trigger a definite plan of action. It may be useful to write out that plan together. When you see signs of stress or other events that point toward renewed mis-eating and weight problems, speak up, gently but firmly, for taking action.

This is a long list of things to do. They are not obligations, but possibilities. View them and the whole program as a resource for the future. You have worked hard and should be congratulated as a partner who has taken a constructive and important step toward solving a problem in your lives together.

APPENDIX

PART I: TRUE OR FALSE

(Give yourself 2 points for each correct answer.)

Circle
Your Answer

1. Learning new self-control skills is more important than the short-term reward of losing pounds. True or False

   T F

2. Recording everything I eat in my food diary is my way of keeping track and of learning to be honest with myself. True or False

   T F

3. A calorie is
   A) a measure of weight of food.
   B) the fat content of a food.
   C) a measure of energy.

   A B C

4. It is not important to note victories in my diary notes because I should only be concerned with why and when I mis-eat. True or False

   T F

5. When I buy a five-ounce piece of beef and cook it, cooked meat will be fairly close to four ounces. True or False

   T F

6. The goal of a calorie-counting system is complete freedom to eat any foods, as long as I monitor the quantity of my intake in a way that will allow me to decrease (or maintain) my weight. True or False   T F

7. Generally, one philosophy of this book is to
   A) lose weight by avoiding high-calorie food.
   B) find a diet that will take the weight off the quickest way.
   C) eat a balanced intake similar to my normal food program.   A B C

8. Whole-grain cereals and breads, potatoes, and dried fruits are high in
   A) fats.
   B) protein.
   C) carbohydrates.   A B C

9. Breakfast is the most important meal of the day. No one should even skip breakfast. True or False   T F

10. Self-control is inborn. Some people have it, some don't. True or False   T F

11. The slower I eat, the more food I'll consume. True or False   T F

12. Once I've decided to diet, I should see if I can do it alone and surprise my friends and relatives. True or False   T F

13. Natural "thinnies" usually can eat anything and as much as they want. True or False   T F

14. Observing the eating habits of thin friends and relatives may be upsetting and should be avoided. True or False   T F

15. To help children to stay or get slim, you should
    A) make them eat three regular meals each day.
    B) let them play with their food.
    C) have them take small portions so they can clean their plates.   A B C

16. Hunger feelings, like sleepiness, tend to wax and wane. They do not get uniformly stronger the longer I postpone eating. True or False   T F

17. A diet is only a temporary solution.
    True or False   T F

18. Scheduling and planning snacks is
    A) a bad habit to get into.
    B) an important technique in solving problem times.
    C) only permissible when the food is very low in calories.   A B C

19. If my body's energy system is perfectly in balance, I am taking in the same amount as I am burning. At the balance point, my weight stays the same. True or False   T F

20. Exercise will increase my appetite.
    True or False   T F

21. When I reach a plateau and don't seem to be able to lose any more weight, a little more activity can make the difference, even at the same calorie-intake level. True or False   T F

22. Exercise is a good antidepressant. Physical activity helps chase away the blues. True or False   T F

23. A walk in the evening after dinner will tend to speed up my metabolism a bit and help me to burn the calories taken in at the meal even faster. True or False   T F

24. Loneliness, fear, or the inability to get active are often confused with boredom.
    True or False   T F

25. Throwing away half of my meal was a shock treatment to enable me to
    A) control stopping eating.
    B) realize the high cost of food.
    C) practice self-denial.   A B C

26. Obese people are often "foodaholics" and should simply eliminate permanently certain foods they can't stop eating. True or False   T F

27. Sometimes, when nothing else works, it's okay to mis-eat. True or False   T F

28. The person who will succeed in permanent weight control is the one who
   A) knows her weaknesses and avoids them.
   B) can stick to a diet.
   C) expects to mis-eat from time to time.   A B C

29. Guilt is useful in improving our control of eating. True or False   T F

30. If I've had a long and costly binge, the best thing is to really starve myself the next day to make up for it. True or False   T F

31. Leaving food on my plate is
   A) always economically wasteful.
   B) important because restaurants often give far too much.
   C) a bad example to set for my children.   A B C

32. Leaving food on my plate will, in the long run, result in saving money and food. True or False   T F

33. If I reach a weight plateau, I should
   A) fast for a week.
   B) temporarily reduce sugar and starches.
   C) delay until I feel more motivated to diet.   A B C

34. Relaxation exercises are important because they give more energy. True or False   T F

35. When I wake up feeling upset or anxious, I should slow down, relax, and plan simple goals that I know I can achieve for the day. True or False   T F

36. It is best to do my grocery shopping right before dinner. True or False   T F

37. Rehearsing with a friend can help me to be more assertive when I am confronted with the actual situation. True or False   T F

38. By asking for what I need, whether it be help or advice, cooperation or affection, I am always increasing my changes of overcoming difficulties and frustrations. True or False   T F

39. The more I put myself first and start to live life my way,
    A) the more problems I'll stir up that I can't solve.
    B) the more selfish I'll become.
    C) the more free I'll be of frustrations that lead to using food as a tranquilizer.   A B C

40. The best way to handle a friend who insists that you join in and eat a high-calorie food with her is to avoid that person until you reach goal weight. True or False   T F

41. Sometimes, banning a food forever because it is so tempting creates a tension that ultimately leads to a binge of the forbidden food.
    True or False   T F

42. When practicing control of a high-temptation food,
    A) take safe situations first.
    B) if the opportunity arises, it's okay to skip to a more dangerous situation.
    C) if you fail, just go on to the next item up on the list.   A B C

43. It shouldn't be necessary to give myself rewards for steps forward. The scale should be reward enough. True or False   T F

44. If eating out is a problem time for me, I should
    A) avoid eating out while dieting.
    B) plan ahead for these occasions by budgeting calories.
    C) go on a fast to make up for mis-eating.   A B C

45. It's important to eat meals on a strict schedule. Discipline is the best route to control. True or False   T   F

46. When eating in a restaurant, it is best to
   A) order à la carte, if possible.
   B) order everything at once.
   C) starve myself several hours before going.   A   B   C

47. It is best to postpone quitting smoking until eating control is well in hand. True or False   T   F

48. When on vacation, it is a good idea to
   A) plan to maintain and not to lose weight.
   B) let loose and take a vacation from calorie counting.
   C) stick to my regime the same as I would if I were at home.   A   B   C

49. Sometimes, changing my entire image to a slim, more attractive person may be a bit scary. It's a natural feeling. True or False   T   F

50. Regaining some weight after successfully reaching my goal means
   A) I'm human and have stresses in my life.
   B) I never really accomplished anything at all.
   C) I might as well just accept being fat.   A   B   C

PART 2: CALORIE KNOWLEDGE

(Give yourself 5 points for each correct answer)

1 cup fresh strawberries	_____
4-oz. portion ground beef	_____
8-oz. glass lowfat milk	_____
½ cup cottage cheese	_____
¼ broiled chicken	_____
1 soft-boiled egg	_____
1 medium apple	_____

1 slice pizza	——————
1 cup peas	——————
1 doughnut	——————
4-oz. portion cooked lamb	——————
1 cup clear broth	——————
4-oz. glass orange juice	——————
1 cup mashed potatoes	——————
1-oz. slice cheese	——————
1 medium tomato	——————
tuna salad sandwich	——————
1 slice bread	——————
1 pat butter	——————
1 taco	——————

(Find the answers to the tests at the end of the Appendices.)

WEEK-TO-WEEK RECORD

Each week, record your Sunday weight and average calories for the week on this form for your own records. Record your measurements once every four weeks.

	Weight	Average Calories (Food)	Upper Arm	Chest	Waist	Hips	Upper Thighs
				MEASUREMENTS			
1							
2							
3							
4							
5							
6							
7							
8							
9							
10							
11							
12							
13							

KNOWLEDGE TEST—ANSWER SHEET

1. True	18. B	35. True
2. True	19. True	36. False
3. C	20. False	37. True
4. False	21. True	38. True
5. True	22. True	39. C
6. True	23. True	40. False
7. C	24. True	41. True
8. C	25. A	42. A
9. False	26. False	43. False
10. False	27. True	44. B
11. False	28. C	45. False
12. False	29. False	46. A
13. False	30. False	47. True
14. False	31. B	48. A
15. B	32. True	49. True
16. True	33. B	50. A
17. True	34. True	

CALORIE-COUNT ANSWERS*

1 cup fresh strawberries	50	4-oz. portion cooked lamb	400
4-oz. portion ground beef	400	1 cup clear broth	50
8-oz. glass lowfat milk	120	4-oz. glass orange juice	50
½ cup cottage cheese	100	1 cup mashed potatoes	250
¼ broiled chicken	100	1-oz. slice cheese	100
1 soft-boiled egg	100	1 medium tomato	30
1 medium apple	70	sandwich	500
1 slice pizza	250	1 slice bread	60
1 cup peas	100	1 pat butter	50
1 doughnut	220	1 taco	350

*Credit yourself with a correct answer if you are within 10 calories. For example, a cup of fresh strawberries is 50. If you answer 40 to 60, give yourself credit for a correct answer.

UNDIET CLUBS

Much could be written about forming and running a group, especially one concerned with the special problems related to weight control. This appendix is intended to serve as a brief guide. Weight control is a difficult, often long-term, problem. Most of us can use help and support. A member-run group is not only a way to reduce the cost of professional assistance, but such a group may prove more effective than the professionally led program. We are in the process of doing research on member-led Undiet Clubs and would welcome feedback from readers on their experience. You can write to Dr. Albert R. Marston at the Psychology Department, University of Southern California, University Park, Los Angeles, CA 90089.

Structure

As we indicated in the Introduction, you can use a number of ways to get started, e.g., announcements of an organizing meeting in newspapers, church bulletins, local radio stations, etc. The organizing meeting can be used to review the proposed organization structure and select a first round of job assignments. If the initial turnout is greater than 15, you should consider more than one group, organized either geographically or by preferred meeting times. Once your area has more than one club, you should be aware of locations, meeting times, and contact people; so that you can refer potential new members who may find it easier to belong to another group. You may want to enlist the help of a local professional to publicize the organization, get things started, and serve as a consultant (dietician, physician, home economist, etc.). However, such assistance is not required to have a successful group.

We mentioned 15 as an optimal size. You certainly can have a larger group but beware of losing contact with one another when you get much over 25. At this point, a split into two groups is probably a good idea. There are a few other issues about membership worth noting, though they may not be problems. Sex: most weight control groups are made up predominantly of women. If you can get a more even mix of men and women, that will prove interesting, perhaps productive, and probably problematic (due to competition of various kinds). You will have to deal with the pros and cons should the situation arise. More common is the problem of the male minority in an almost all female group. Other sometimes touchy subjects in groups are age and weight range. The latter can especially breed friction: very overweight members resent the slightly overweight person who may, in fact, experience all the same eating problems, but without some of the social ones. As much as possible, we recommend that such problems be brought out in the open and discussed. See if you can say clearly to one another, "These are differences we can't resolve, only recognize, but we may be able to live with them and even find help from the members with very different backgrounds and problems." Such a statement can eventually become part of a club credo which can be copied and given to all members (with such other principles as, "no gossiping, no personal attacks, we're all responsible to contribute effort to the club and one another").

A person should visit once before becoming a member and know what he/she is getting into. Membership should be open and not involve votes. But, the new member probably should make a clear commitment to join, e.g., signing the credo, agreeing to attendance or notifying the appropriate person, stating goals as to weight loss, agreeing to share duties, etc.

Two types of members present special problems: the dropout and the person who reaches goal weight. We suggest that you set up a telephone chain; so that every member gets a call every week (or before every meeting, if you decide to meet less often). This will serve as a reminder, a way of supporting each other between meetings, and a way of tracking dropouts. Some people are clear-cut dropouts; they will say definitely that they're no longer interested. Most potential dropouts fade slowly, missing more and more meetings, promising to return, and eventually disappearing. Try to make clear that losing weight is not a criterion for membership, that people who are at a plateau or even gaining will not be exposed or ridiculed, and that problem periods are the most important times to get the help of the group. So, it should be part of the group's philosophy to keep after lagging members and urge them to bring problems to the group.

People who reach goal weight have a natural tendency to drop out of support systems, wanting to believe that they are "cured" and will never need help again. Every group should do its best to keep such members, for three reasons: they *will* need help, they can be an example and a help to others, and the process of helping others will firm up their own commitment to maintain. They can be given special status, honor, and roles to keep them involved.

There are three aspects of club structure which should be agreed on as soon as possible: dues, meeting pattern, and job assignments. It may be best to operate without dues as much as possible, collecting donations for specific needs as they arise. If regular costs develop (room rental, printing), then a small fee may have to be collected. We recommend weekly meetings of about two hours, either in various members' houses or at free community facilities. For obvious reasons, refreshments should not be served (with an exception discussed below), though some simple beverage can help before meetings start and during breaks. Meeting rooms should, if possible, be arranged in a semi-circle with the leader, or facilitator at the open end. It's important that people face one another as much as possible. Each group will have to decide by consensus how to handle the perennial problem of smoking. A good strategy is to limit smoking to outside the room during a 10-minute break midway through the meeting when everyone should be urged to stretch and move around (but reconvene promptly).

We feel that it is vital that all members have a regular job in the functioning of the club, and that these jobs be rotated as frequently as once a month. Involvement is essential. Here is a brief list of possible jobs; many of their functions will be clearer after reading the section on meeting procedure: meeting leader, back-up leader, meeting arranger, meeting recorder, historian (membership lists, assignment lists, etc.), treasurer, telephone coordinator, new member advisor, special programs and guest speaker coordinator, referral service, presenter, weight recorder, public action coordinator, idea and recipe exchange, *The Undiet* reference person. It's no accident that the list totals 15, the optimum group size we recommended.

Meeting Procedure

We think that it helps the stability and effectiveness of the group to have a regular and fairly structured meeting routine. The one suggested below has worked well for various kinds of groups; you can adopt your own version.

1. WEIGH-IN. The weight recorder should bring a reasonably accurate bathroom scale and spend the first 15 minutes *privately* weighing in each member who has a card containing name, goal weight, and weights for each meeting date. One of your first group decisions will be to decide whether each member should keep and bring his/her own card, or whether the weight recorder should keep all the cards in a file box. If confidentiality is kept, the latter system has some advantages: the member feels that someone else knows his/her weight, increasing a sense of responsibility; and the club has an overall record of performance. We do not recommend reading out weight losses or gains, or any other form of overt reward or punishment. The group should be a learning resource and a general support network, not dependent on weight fluctuations. That way you get the advantage of the group, while retaining the importance of individual freedom and responsibility.

2. INTRODUCTION. Every attendee should say his/her name to facilitate name recognition and allow the historian to keep track of attendance.

3. ASSIGNMENT REVIEW. If the group is proceeding through *The Undiet*, as described below, there will be periodic tasks for members to do in connection with the chapter(s) covered in the preceding meeting. In addition, an individual may, as a result of the group discussion, decide to try a particular technique to solve a problem. The meeting recorder for the previous meeting should have a list of those commitments to be reviewed at the next

meeting. The assignment review should be simple, brief and non-judgmental. Simply go around the room and have everyone report whether they tried the activity, whether it worked, and what ideas they have about it. This should take about 15 minutes.

This is a good point to mention a meeting technique which we feel all clubs of this type should adopt: *No judgments, no cross-talk.* When someone reports, there should be no comment. The only discussion should be in the problem-solving phase of the meeting. The leader may have to occasionally cut off a speaker, especially if he/she is in some way attacking another member. Usually a private reminder after the meeting can solve this kind of problem.

4. PROBLEM-SOLVING.   Each member should have the opportunity to present a problem to the group. To conserve time and help the shy, we recommend that sheets of paper be available during the weigh-in time for people to write about a problem and submit it to the meeting recorder who reads aloud each problem to open it for discussion. Ideally, the sheets should have a space for name, date, statement of problem, and possible solutions (to be filled in during the discussion). If you can get those office forms that have attached carbon copy, the member can go home with a plan and the historian can have a copy for assignment review at the next meeting (when that copy too is returned to the member). All members should be urged to submit problems at least once a month.

When a problem has been read aloud, the leader should focus the group's attention first on understanding the problem; i.e., simply asking the person questions (when, where, with whom does that happen; what have you tried; etc.?).* When the problem seems clear, the leader can open the discussion for brainstorming, listing as many strategies as people can think of. *The Undiet* reference person is important here, to have the book at hand and try to suggest chapters or pages that are relevant to the problem. After

*Leading a meeting is an art every member can learn with practice. A shy leader may want to have the backup leader (available for emergency absence of designated leader) act as co-leader, sharing the front of the room and the coordination of the discussion. A good resource for learning about meetings is a book called *How to Make Meetings Work*, by Michael Doyle and David Strauss (New York: Wyden Books, 1976).

that the person whose problem is being discussed should indicate which strategies he or she intends to try that week. The recorder can write these down and give the copy to the member as a form of contract to try something new during the coming week. All members should be urged to bring notebooks and pens to jot down ideas or assignments. All members should also have a membership list kept updated by the historian.

The leader will have to judge time for each problem, based on the number and types submitted. This whole section should last about half an hour. Some problems may have to be postponed, or problems selected randomly for discussion. The member whose problem is not discussed should be contacted after the meeting or by phone by *The Undiet* reference person who can at least provide some input about the problem. The leader must also judge if a problem should not be brought up. Problems should relate to weight control. Other personal problems may inevitably be mentioned, but the leader should recommend, privately, that other problems be brought to other resources. Here the Referral Service member should be available with a list of resources to give the member, privately outside the meeting.

5. NEW MATERIAL. The *presenter* for the week should spend 15-30 minutes describing the material in the chapter(s) scheduled for the coming week, answering questions, and making assignments clear.* Depending on the topic for the week, the presenter should try to end the presentation with a group activity suggested by the material (e.g., everyone bring an apple to eat slowly and sensuously, practice muscle relaxation and imagery, a calorie or portion size test, review of restaurant menus for calorie values).

6. SHARING AND PLANS FOR NEXT MEETING. The last 15 minutes should be reserved for members to share ideas or feelings. Again, there should be no cross-talk and there should be a clear reminder at each meeting that there is to be no gossiping afterwards about what is said. Any ideas, recipes, or resources a

---

*As an alternative, the presenter could play one of the audiotapes from our series *Comprehensive Weight Control*, available from BMA, 200 Park Ave. South, New York, NY 10003.

member would like to share could also be written on a card to be kept in an idea file by the person currently responsible for the *Idea and Recipe Exchange* which would be available for browsing before and after each meeting. Before the close of the meeting, the leader and historian should clarify who is responsible for various tasks, especially arrangements for the next meeting. The telephone coordinator should assign everyone someone else to phone before the next meeting (including those not present), to see if they can be of any help to that person and to remind him/her of the next meeting. If anyone has a special program or guest speaker to suggest, he/she should agree to work with that coordinator to set it up. As with all matters of procedure or program, decisions should be made by consensus, avoiding divisive debate and voting whenever possible.

An important part of this segment of the meeting, and as an occasional main topic for presentation, is the work of the *Public Action Coordinator(s)*. The problem of overweight and nutrition is a public as well as a personal one. The promotion of high calorie food (especially for children), unavailability of nutrition information, lack of physical recreation resources, and many other public matters contribute to the problems faced by the overweight and formerly overweight. Combatting these public problems is not only a service but helps the overweight person blame him/herself less and devote energy outwards. Petitions for better food in schools, lobbying for better recreation resources, public exposure of nutritionally unhealthful products, and many other action techniques are available to the club. This is an area that members who have reached goal weight might be especially suited to coordinate.

Meeting Content

The Undiet Club is designed to be a support group which uses this book as a structure to study and solve the problems related to weight control. While there is plenty of room for flexibility, we would like to suggest a sequence which may help to organize the content of the meetings and the learning experience of the members. Although some clubs could be closed groups (i.e., organized at one time to go through the process together), we envision most as ongoing and open to new members. The sequence can be stretched as needed to accommodate guest speakers, or the group's need to slow down (e.g., to catch up on a backlog of individual problems).

1. ORGANIZATION MEETING. Someone or some group has gotten the club together for the first time. The points in this appendix can be reviewed, modified, and a structure agreed on. Initial assignment of tasks and arrangements for at least one more meeting are made. People will be in varying situations as to weight, current diet, and knowledge about the book. To coordinate a starting framework, everyone should agree to read (or review) chapters 1–3 for the next meeting. Perhaps two people who are more experienced with the book will agree to be *The Undiet* reference person and the new member advisor for the next few weeks. Other members can phone either of these people for any help needed with the content of Chapters 1–3. In general, if any newcomer joins the club when the members are working on later chapters, he or she is asked to read Chapters 1–3, get started on the issue of diet and diary keeping and consult with the new member advisor for help. Once past Chapters 1–3, the newcomer can fit in quickly by reading the chapters out of sequence, fitting the reading to the chapters currently being studied by the group.

2. The second meeting can focus on Chapters 2 and 3 in the presentation of new material. The presenter and leader should make sure that all members are clear on such "Undiet" issues as: selecting a diet (or not), whether to use professional help (which is quite compatible with being in an Undiet Club), keeping a diary, and use of partner activities. In general, it is not suggested that non-overweight partners attend Undiet Club meetings. However, when Chapter 14 is the topic, you may want to add a meeting to get input from partners and discuss problems (related to weight control!).

3. After Chapters 2 and 3 have been covered (you may decide to add an extra meeting on these two chapters), each meeting can focus on a chapter, proceeding from 4 through 16.

4. After Chapter 16 has been discussed, hold a review meeting (with the presenter using Chapter 17 as a focus). Members can discuss where they stand in their own progress toward (or maintaining) a goal weight. The group can review itself as an organization and discuss changes for the future. Again, this review may take more than one meeting. It may involve the decision to split into two groups, each wih somewhat different goals.

5. Start the cycle over again with a presentation of Chapter 2 and discussion of motivation. Depending on the composition of the group, the succeeding cycles can be a repetition of the first one; as you learn and change, the material in the chapters will have new meaning and new ideas will emerge in discussion. Or, you may decide, if most members have covered the whole book, to insert more guest speakers or discussions on new topics; or to devote more of the meetings to the Problem Solving section.

With the cooperation and effort of the members and frequent rotation of assignments, this cycle can repeat indefinitely. Emphasis will change with new members or a predominance of maintenance members. When enough of the group has reached goal weight, you may want to urge several maintenance members to form a separate group and to recruit and help new people.

We hope this brief Appendix helps you on your way to forming and enjoying an *Undiet Club*. Please contact us with any questions or feedback about your experience.

SELECTED READINGS

ALBERTI, R. E. and M. L. EMMONS. *Your Perfect Right: A Guide To Assertive Behavior,* 2nd ed. Chicago: Impact Press, 1974.

BERLAND, T. *Rating The Diets.* New York: Consumer Guide, Signet Books, 1980.

BLOOM, L. Z., K. COBURN, and J. PEARLMAN. *The New Assertive Woman.* New York: Dell, 1976.

BRUCH, H. *Eating Disorders: Obesity, Anorexia And The Person Within.* New York: Basic Books, 1973.

ELLIS, A., and Q. A. HARPER. *A New Guide To Rational Living.* Englewood Cliffs, N.J.: Prentice-Hall, 1975.

GOTTMAN, J., C. NOTARIUS, J. CONSO, and H. MARKHAM. *A Couple's Guide To Communication.* Champaign, Ill.: Research Press, 1976.

KRAUS, B. *The Dictionary Of Calories And Carbohydrates.* New York: Plume Books, 1973.

LEWINSOHN, P., R. MUNOZ, M. YOUNGREN, and A. ZEISS. *Control Your Depression.* Englewood Cliffs, N.J.: Prentice-Hall, 1978.

MAYER, J. *A Diet For Living.* New York: David McKay Co., Inc., 1975.

MILLER, W. and R. MUNOZ. *How To Control Your Drinking.* Englewood Cliffs, N.J.: Prentice-Hall, 1973.

INDEX

215